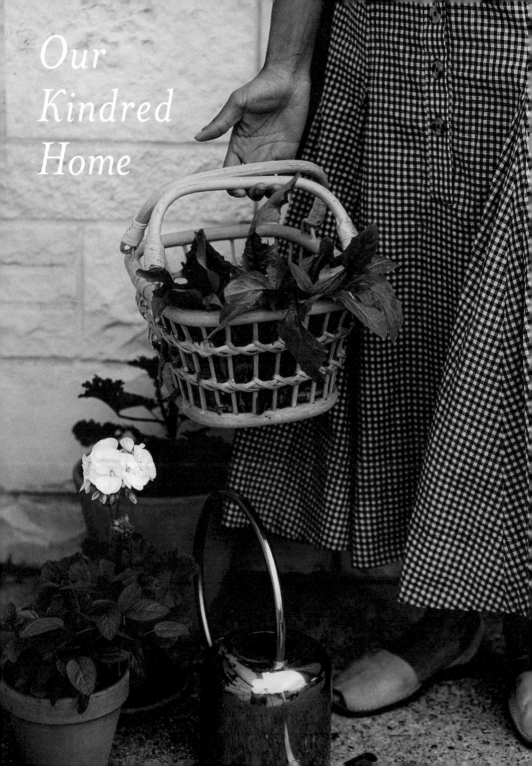

Our Kindred Home

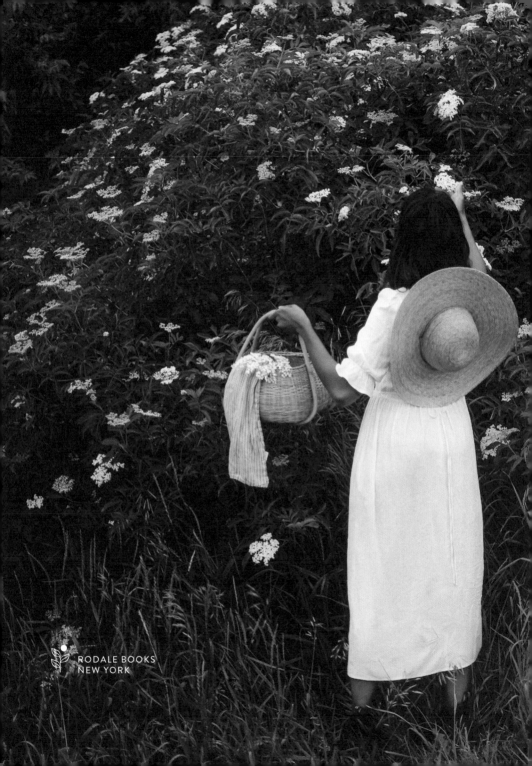

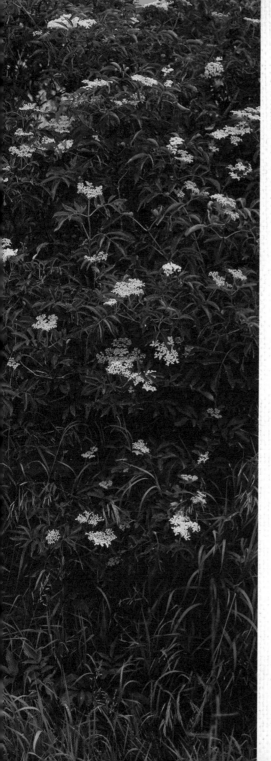

HERBAL RECIPES,
PLANT WISDOM &
SEASONAL RITUALS
FOR REKINDLING
CONNECTION WITH
THE EARTH

Our
Kindred
Home

ALYSON MORGAN

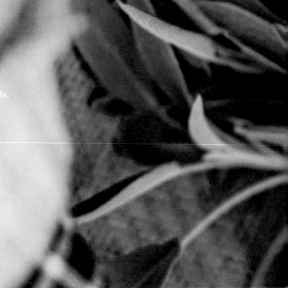

To Magnolia, my moon, and Griffin, my sun,
the ancestors, my stars. You are my guiding lights.

To the bird, the bloom, the earthworm, and bee.
To the human and more than kin we share this
Earth with, may we remember the ease, the joy,
and wholeness of being connected.

Published in the United States by Rodale Books, an imprint of Random House, a division of Penguin Random House LLC, New York.
RodaleBooks.com
RandomHouseBooks.com

RODALE and the Plant colophon are registered trademarks of Penguin Random House LLC.

Library of Congress Cataloging-in-Publication Data
Names: Morgan, Alyson, author.
Title: Our kindred home: herbal recipes, plant wisdom, and seasonal rituals for rekindling connection with the Earth / Alyson Morgan.
Description: First edition. | New York: Rodale Books, 2023. | Includes bibliographical references and index.
Identifiers: LCCN 2022034041 | ISBN 9780593235980 (hardcover) | ISBN 9780593235997 (ebook)
Subjects: LCSH: Herbs—Therapeutic use. | Herbs—Utilization.
Classification: LCC RM666.H33 M656 2023 | DDC 615.3/21—dc23/eng/20220912
LC record available at https://lccn.loc.gov/2022034041

ISBN 978-0-593-23598-0
Ebook ISBN 978-0-593-23599-7

Printed in China

Book cover and interior design by Jen Wang
Principal photography by Alyson Morgan
Photographs on pages 6, 12, 50–51, 92, 100, 115, and 122 by Karlee Mikkelson
Illustrations by Frances Rehmann

10 9 8 7 6 5 4 3 2 1

First Edition

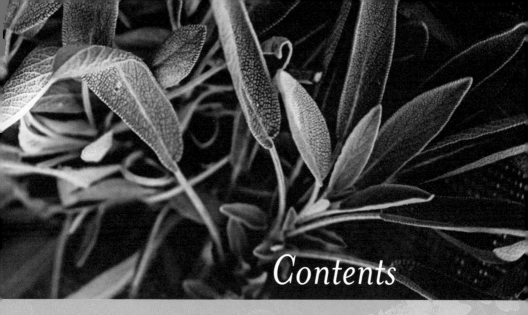

Contents

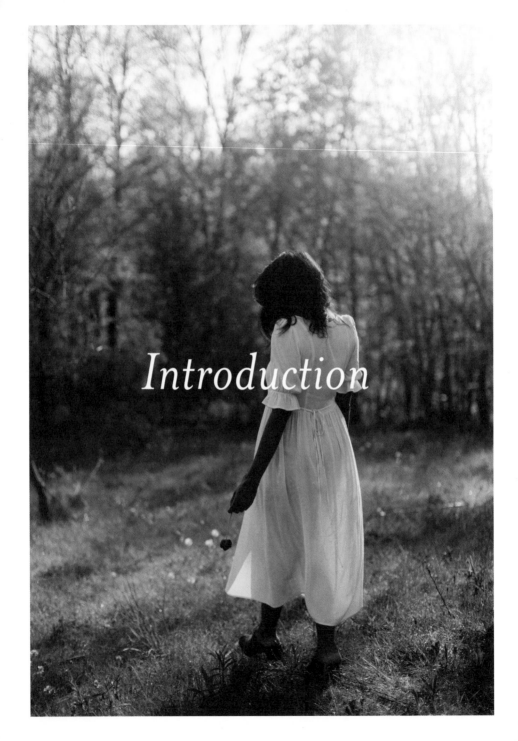

Introduction

*M*uch like the living world around us, our bodies are complex ecosystems, home to water, fire, earth, wind, and spirit.

Emotions swell. Like waves on the brink of cresting, rising within my body, carrying old stories, old feelings. When my emotional waters have been calm for some time, the rising tide of self-hatred is the one that can take me under so quickly. I gasp for air at the thought that I can even hold such loathing for myself. I found that, much like a riptide, fighting the wave makes it harder, so I must ride it out. I used to wholeheartedly believe the stories these swells tell and take them for truths. I know now the true origins come from a dark and ancient sea not of my own making, a sea not unlike the one that carried my ancestors in the belly of a ship. Understanding its origin does not make it any easier to *feel*, but it does make it easier to not be wholly engulfed. Life contains mystery felt yet unseen that we cannot quite comprehend.

My buoy in this sea of darkness is joy. The stars and the moon are anchors outside of myself, whispering, "You do not travel alone; when you are lost, we can be your guide." I'm learning to allow my emotions to fully surface, letting the salt water of my tears cleanse me. The only way through is to feel. When I began to listen attentively and value my own inklings, it opened a new world and allowed me to rebuild a relationship of trust within and the ability to discern information in the outside world. My unlearning and relearning began when I started listening to plants.

I never understood the gravity of heaviness and pain I carried in my brown body in this white-dominated society. I don't think my mother quite understood it either. Why was I so sensitive and so affected? More than emotionality, I felt something deep in my bones and blood. Gifted and woven together by the threads of my diverse ancestry, known and unknown, Afro Indigenous, Haitian, European, place, stories, and languages are sown into me. The threads of my ancestries span continents and oceans. My body is the keeper of their stories and the pain of both the colonizers and the enslaved. Nestled between sinew, nerve, and tendon, I hold acute pain of being stolen from homelands and concurrently dogged resilience of surviving it all. We all, undoubtedly, hold more than we are aware of.

Our bodies are our primary and sacred vessels for the time we travel here on Earth. From the moment we are born, our first language is our senses. The vibration of our mother's heartbeat is the first we experience, the warmth of the skin, the taste of milk, and from those very moments we begin to process information about the world around us. Is it safe, am I loved, am I fed, are my bodily needs met? We learn from these first moments, through sensory information, for months and years of our lives before we learn language. It informs how our nervous systems and our brains become wired.

I was loved, fed, and held, yet my own pain was brought to light in a car accident in high school. Physical trauma laid bare emotional trauma. With my corporeal vessel cracked open, the light poured through my wounds, and this trial became my initiation. I could have died at sixteen years old, but I see it as the day I was born. At this tender age, I was made aware how precious and fleeting our lives in these human bodies are. We are here for a blip on the timescale. That accident changed me physically, spiritually, and mentally. I wanted to live my life to the fullest now that I knew how short life could be, but I felt stifled by toxic relationships to myself, my body, and to people around me. A deep sense of disconnection haunted me.

Throughout my journey, I've learned how much trauma is stored within my body. This unprocessed trauma caused nervous system dysregulation, triggered by continuing racial and cultural wounding. To truly begin on a path of healing, I needed to find safe space and ways to ease my nervous system and befriend what I was carrying. I found safe space in the garden and a nostalgic ease with the natural world. I am grateful for years of access to mental health resources, body work, and somatic practices. Yet there is so much wisdom and healing to be gleaned from daily rituals and deep connection with plants. I've learned safe ways to ground myself into the soil of my being. Plants are a catalyst for deeper healing, and when they were woven into my daily practices, I found a sense of balance and ease. There are so many resources out there that teach us the constituents of plants and their biochemical processes, but I want to return to the root of plant connection. Our ancestors connected with embodied awareness and practices to form relationships with plants to weather storms, for seasons of lack and abundance, incorporating that relationship into simple yet sacred daily practices for nourishment, healing, resilience, and community care. So many of us have lost that knowledge and in turn are lost.

This book is about plants because plants want to be our guides through this season of humanity here on earth. Plants are our ancestors, and they want us to recollect and retell their stories and to weave them into our lives. I want to convey the intimacy, serendipity, and magic I've found in my relationship with the natural world, because connecting to the spirit of more than human beings is healing.

A plant isn't just a plant. Plants are the basis of our food, homes, clothing, and medicine. In these times of great chaos, plants are reaching out for kinship, whether in the forest, cultivated on your windowsill, or growing outside your office window. There is deep nourishment for our nervous systems and relationships available to be called into service. When I became too overwhelmed with the awareness of my own trauma, of my ancestral and intergenerational pain, the struggle of living in a Black female body in a white supremacist society, and my own internalized feelings of inferiority, the antidote was somatic awareness through yoga, attending to my body's wants and needs, and a deep listening to plants. Chamomile helps me rest and digest. Tulsi's scent immediately grounds me when I'm panicking and trying to navigate the climate crisis with two young children. Lavender lets me know in this present moment that serenity is safe. The solution for me has been to slow down, to cultivate awareness in what's happening in my body, to connect to the seasonal and cyclical shifts around me, and to incorporate the plants in simple, comforting, nourishing yet meaningful ways throughout my days to remember the joy of being alive.

From a warm beverage on a cool, crisp fall morning to a cooling herbal shrub in the oppressive heat of summer, herbal steams for spring allergies, or a lavender dessert to ease social anxiety and create an environment of relaxation for friends and folk gathering at your table, plants help us find ease. Some days it only takes a woodland walk to ground me into the present moment; other weeks, nettle infusions pull me up and out of the slog and doldrums of depression.

Not only do plants offer us immediate sensual support, but the knowledge of the plants in our immediate environment helps us connect in deeper ways to our ecosystems and can provide resilience in changing social and ecological landscapes. Do you know which plants aid with wound cleansing and healing, what plant underfoot can soothe a bee sting? Do you know what leaf can help with diarrhea? These are folkways our grandmothers and grandfathers knew, and in cultivating that knowledge, we can build somatic resilience and pass on folk traditions for survival.

The right relationship with the natural world teaches us lessons of reciprocity, of uncertainty, of our true interconnectedness. I share my personal reflections with you out of my greatest hope that plant wisdom can help you on your own journey of understanding yourself, your place, and your ability to process what life circumstances come your way.

We are living in a time of an unveiling, of the collective uncovering of systems of great harm, of destruction, and of exploitation. Colonialism, oppression, racism, and systematic disconnection from nature have existed here for centuries, informing our bodies, passed down from generation to generation. We bear the scars on our hearts, bodies, spirits, and our earth.

There are things we can no longer collectively sweep under the rug. Our human experience can feel wholly overwhelming. Our nervous systems are overloaded, and our responses vary from numbed, escapist, denial, and disassociation. But we cannot run— our lives, I believe, depend on staying and confronting all we've shoved down into the depths of our collective unconscious. Plants can help us create safe space to process, to find joy, and to transmute our personal, collective, and ancestral trauma. In the journey into the depths of our experience, we can mine pearls of wisdom to bring back to the surface of our experience to find more joy and levity.

This book is broken into three parts. Part One is a deep and sometimes heavy dive into personal and collective wounds. Part Two discusses how cultivating a relationship with plants can help our disconnection and dis-ease. Part Three lays out recipes, rituals, and rhythms to cultivate wisdom and reclaim joy through earth and season. As you make your way through Part One, I invite you to be mindful of your physical awareness. How the information and stories land in your own body. How the information and stories included might reflect your experience or be something completely new. I know my experience is my own and may be very different from yours, but I believe we have a good deal to learn from each other and our kindred earth when we can learn to listen. Throughout the book, I invite you to mark your page, close the book, and step outside.

I write this for my children, Magnolia and Griffin, so that one day they may be ancestors, and for their children's children, so they may know I endeavored to use my voice for them, speaking a spell for our continued existence. At the time of writing this book, the science indicates we have eleven years to take decisive action on climate change to prevent catastrophic damage. As the earth warms and inaction takes root, this number is dwindling. Humans need to make an urgent shift to avert catastrophic ecological changes, yet some are still debating and arguing whether or not it is real. I cannot wrap my mind around the disconnect. But then I remember we are so coddled in the bubbles of our own lives. We are disconnected from our own personal navigation systems and apt to believe whatever the news and outside sources tell us. I think we all, in one way or another, experience the dis-ease.

We are taught to fear the "other," to dominate each other with the understanding that the earth is ours for the taking. These fallacies underpin our built worlds. Settler colonialism and capitalism beget endless cycles of overconsumption that have systematically severed human relationships with the earth and, in turn, with ourselves. When we are so deeply ungrounded, adrift, wrapped up in our own storylines, and tethered to outdated and harmful ways of being, we cannot see beyond. Yet we must learn to look beyond to plan, prepare, and take right action.

We are currently facing a time unlike any other in human history. We cannot continue to operate cut off from ourselves, the natural world, our ancestors, and each other if we want to survive. To be able to listen and navigate the challenges and be open to the possibilities the next fifty years will present, we need to cultivate the ability to listen, to process, and to work out what lives in our bodies. We must learn to befriend what is carried on our shoulders, the grief we hold in our hearts, the misinformed beliefs we perpetuate. As a Black woman living within white American society, I carry trauma, anxiety, and fears that other people may not carry. Our personal experiences, our ancestral lineages, our stories and minds mean we all have different personal maps and cartographies we bring to the table. Understanding ourselves means we can function in our world in more conscious ways. And these times are calling us all to act and show up in our own lives to transform the effects of human-led climate chaos.

This book has been difficult to write at times, because I want to share my truth as I see and understand it, but my story exists within the global context. My journey to plants does not exist in a vacuum. Plants are political. Many Indigenous people around the world have had to fight for the right to grow their own seeds and retain ownership over their lands in the face of global capitalism. While speaking up and using my voice has been a personal struggle for me, I am not alone. My ancestors whisper at my back, "It's now or never." This book is meant to be a spoonful of honey to help the bitter medicine of reality go down a little easier.

In this book, I explore my experiences and how my path toward healing my body put me in deep connection with the earth. Through plant medicine, I found not only a deep physical healing but a mental, emotional, and spiritual portal to greater awareness of our human and plant ancestors. This book is my attempt to share what I've woven together in my own life and the perspectives I've cultivated over time and through experience. I hope it serves as a starting point, a resource, a guidebook for your own personal reflection and as a little encouragement to those looking to rekindle connection and take on the rooted, decolonized healing work our world desperately craves. To help you in that journey, you'll find more than forty plant monographs, healing seasonal recipes, and rhythms for finding healing with earth and season. Our solutions to the climate crisis will need to be multipronged approaches, not just logic and new technology but working with our hands: embodiment practices, breathing, pulling weeds, walking in the woods, making the bread, tending to the soil, singing to our bones, and loving each other.

Our perspectives on ourselves and each other need a profound shift and dose of love if we are to find healing, with wellness occurring not in singularity but interwoven in the actions, stories, intentions, and support we experience. Wellness feels to me like an integration of my parts, honoring my own inner cycles and seasons.

Wellness encompasses the physical, the emotional, intellectual, social, spiritual, environmental, and occupational. I'm not interested in furthering a colonized view of wellness that is hinged on perfectionism—trying to achieve a perfect state of health or the perfect body—but on embracing wellness as the work to divest from systems of domination, extraction, and global capitalism and invest in relationships and reciprocity. We can heal when we experience and embody our wholeness, our dualities and multiplicities, our light and shadow, pain and joy and share it with others.

We have been exploiting our Earth, objectifying the waters, the soils, the forests, and oceans as resources rather than acknowledging it is the source. We need to embody this shift to fulfill our duty as stewards of the land. If we can remember our place within the web of life, if we can rekindle our intuition and deeper relationship with Earth, it will activate us to improve our response to the climate crisis unfolding before us.

Reclamation

*A practice of reclaiming disparate and unknown
parts of myself.*

I need you to know how beautiful our Earth is to me.

---

*G*rowing up in Northern California, I was gifted an appreciation for the nature around me, absorbed by its beauty. My dad took every opportunity he had when he wasn't working to get us outside and explore. Growing up in apartments, I didn't have a garden, but the dramatic, untouched landscapes and plant life of California, viewed out the car window on hour-long commutes to and from school, are forever transcribed into my heart and mind. The rolling hills dotted with grandfather oak trees were the subjects of my childhood paintings and doodles, the majestic and ancient redwood forests indelibly sketched in my young memory. After camping in the redwoods and awakening to a coastal fog hugging their bark, I knew I was a part of something much greater than myself. As young children with open minds and hearts, we know the sun, the moon, the sky, the wind, the water, and the earth are all eternal medicine.

The beauty of this Earth is unseen mycelia under our feet beneath the mossy forest floor, carrying the whispers of swaying trees between each other. Are they speaking of your presence? It is in the air as the birds carry messages on their wings and the stars guide us home. We are woven into a constellation of living magic. This natural beauty is a portal to healing and affirmation that life deserves our joy and undivided attention. The imperceptible magic of the natural world, the spirit that binds us together, and the creativity running through our veins is hard to explain, and it should not be ignored.

I've been drawn to beauty from a young age. It is a passion of mine, given to me by my father as he taught me how to observe and record a subject, the way the light flickered off a human eye, how to translate the dancing colors I saw onto paper and communicate what

I sensed to another person. Today, photography takes the place of pencil and paper for me, but it is the same act of devotion to the love, the beauty, and the natural world around me. I've often wondered if we could just stop, observe, and worship the gifts of the natural world, to value it wholly, whether this could be enough to comprehend our deep love, interdependence, and reliance on our Earth enough to galvanize us to protect it.

Somewhere along the way, I began to feel an unknown rumbling and quaking inside of me that I didn't understand. I valued beauty but I didn't understand that the other side of that coin was grief. A sea of grief too vast, too complex for my own mind to begin to decipher. In my pain, I foraged for the elements to make sense of myself, my emotions, my body in this world. I was a Black girl in a white-dominated society. I dutifully internalized white supremacy while attending mostly white schools, reinforced by wounding insinuations about what my blackness meant, my value, and my place. It didn't come naturally to me, but I was educated to hate myself and my "blue black skin" darkened by the summer sun. To this day, when I gaze upon my sun-kissed reflection after long days spent out in my garden, it is my practice to kindly dismiss the colonized voice in my head and whisper, "I love you."

Part and parcel, I developed an eating disorder in high school, bingeing and purging almost every meal I ate, trying to find my place among the stick-thin bodies around me and what I consumed from the media. I squeezed my developing curves into skinny jeans, trying to prove my worth and confirm my lovability. Because the standards of beauty were white-centric, I was convinced I was an inferior being. I thought I could never feel better, be accepted, because I could never be white. It's painful to recollect all the ways I was bewildered and dominated, denying myself love and hurting myself. You do not have to be Black to feel the pain and restriction white supremacy inflicts on the mind and spirit. I share this story because I find healing in my vulnerability. We all suffer in our own ways, but we do not have to do so in isolation.

In college, I changed my major from art to international relations. I inched closer to my wound, my roots, to locate my experience in the global context as a first-generation Haitian American on my mother's side. She rarely spoke of her first home, but as part of the diaspora, I had an unquenchable longing for a place I never knew or called home.

Throughout my time in academia, I came face-to-face with tumultuous depths within. I experienced a sudden depression studying the colonization of Africa, the history of Haiti's slave rebellion, and the centuries of international intervention meant to keep the descendants of the world's only successful slave rebellion in subjugation. This is where my root work began. I experienced high levels of social anxiety when I was working and presenting with white peers, constantly feeling less than and questioning my own self-worth. Why was I one of only 1,138 black students in a student population of 30,000 at a large public university? I engaged in toxic relationships and compulsive spending and did not set boundaries, believing I wasn't worth it.

I remember reading the work of Franz Fanon for the first time in a course entitled Colonialism in Africa. Little did I know I was going to be confronting my own "colonized mind," and I remember the fog of realization and not being able to see straight for a week—dazed, confused, and feeling like my life and identity were a lie.

Essentially, my degree utilized different lenses of varying subjects, paradigms, and pedagogies in the fields of anthropology, history, sociology, and political sciences to examine the phenomenon of colonialism, its extension in the capitalist system, and the effects on people and the planet. Our health, our natural resources, our livelihood, our cultures, and climate—I learned we are all endangered by imperial colonial capitalist systems run rampant, in the form of wars, waste, and famines. Many of our ancestors and many people today are oppressed by these interlocking systems.

What I didn't understand at first was why these classes, the readings, and the questions we were examining were having such a profound effect on my mental health. Why are women around the world systematically disadvantaged? What are the driving forces behind agricultural industrialization? Why are the waterways and our bodies being polluted with petrochemicals? I began to see the woven interconnectedness of so many of the world's problems. I was gaining an intellectual understanding of my felt experience, my ancestral lineage, and it led me to a nervous breakdown. I wasn't just studying a topic: I was seeing the root of my own wounding laid bare.

I eventually found a therapist, withdrew from graduate school, and was just treading water, mentally and emotionally. Apart from my studies, I was actively engaged in political activism on our college campus. And I fell in love. It was at this intersection of passionate expression that I claimed my voice, located safe spaces to process and an outlet for the ancient rage I felt bubbling under the surface at the face of injustice. But in this season of love and war, fighting felt unsustainable and without tangible results. I was drained and needed to reclaim a sense of joy and wonder. The world was a dark place—I knew this in my bones. I needed to reclaim the relationship to the light in myself.

My partner, AJ, and I decided to leave academia and move to the Midwest. In order to continue my healing and learning to care for myself, I enrolled in a yoga teacher training. I had done yoga or asanas since I was in high school, often in the solitude of my bedroom, because there wasn't a proliferation of yoga studios at the time. Yoga as both a physical and spiritual practice helped me embrace my body as a worthy vessel and yoke my mind and body into wholeness. I didn't realize, until I was on the mat, all the ways I dissociated to cope. Teacher training was an investment in my worth and inherent value. I was still struggling, after uprooting and moving from a racially and culturally diverse upbringing in California to the predominantly white and segregated city of Milwaukee. I was having anxieties in social spaces, experiencing subtle racism and sexism in the workplace, and felt so far away from the comforts of family and home. I had to find my grounding. Slowly but surely, these experiences began to move through my body.

And then motherhood came calling. In motherhood, I understood my body was a vessel for more than just myself. It was life giving. The weight of my choices and decisions was paramount. What I put in my body, what I put on my body, and my values became more than about me. Through motherhood, I realized the importance of what I learned in school, and I was able to separate out the trinkets of wisdom and gain perspective from the traumas I held. As I cradled my daughter, Magnolia, in my arms, a fire in my heart began to burn. A fierce burning, reminiscent of the passion I felt chanting in solidarity at marches and protests. I had to protect her and this place we now both called home. This is when I began to feel called to share my voice through writing. In birthing my daughter, I birthed a new version of myself. Shaky and unsure, I started to hear a little whisper inside myself become a little louder. A mother's intuition was my own intuition, a voice that I hadn't heard in my life for some time: an inner compass.

As my intuition grew louder, AJ and I decided our path was taking us in a different direction, a lifestyle different from our own upbringing, a slower pace, in a place neither of us had ever lived. We decided to leave the familiar chaos and anxiety of city living to move to a small rural town in the Midwest. Me, a Black woman from Northern California in the middle of Midwestern Wisconsin. I was scared out of my mind. It didn't make much sense on paper, but I was compelled to listen to those whispers growing louder. I didn't know it at the time, but it was this move that enabled me to reclaim and heal through rooting into place. We downsized and purchased a small cottage owned by an herbalist. It was here in the herb garden that I began to hear the plants loud and clear. I wanted to nurture the garden, to homestead and learn new skills, to learn how to grow our own food and flowers, to grow our resilience against climate uncertainty, but what I found in the garden was more than I could ever have imagined.

In embracing my inner whispers and my inner knowing, my journey brought me to the plants, to myself and my ancestors. In slowing down, in leaving behind the comforts of what I knew and what I thought I wanted, I could hear myself. With the plants, the soil, the moon, the birdsong, the earthworms, and my children running barefoot in the garden, I re-mothered myself. The plants created a safety I'd never really known; they held my nervous system and made it okay to confront and sit with my anxiety, fears, doubts, and ancestral trauma, and to learn to love it all.

I share my story because I believe humans are carrying worlds upon worlds and wounds upon wounds inside their bodies, some born out of their personal experiences, relationships, traumas and some from our families, our ancestral lineages, stories we didn't live in this life but carry in our cells. The pace of capitalism and our everyday anxieties, lack of access to mental health, and lack of safety, all add up to mean we are not processing our experiences, our emotions and our traumas. Our burdens and our resilience are woven into our being. We don't have to live from our wounds but can live from our joy, and the plants can show us how.

Land Acknowledgment,
Ancestral Practices, Shadow Work

When we learn to take the time to process our fears, our failures, and our vulnerability, it grows our capacity for compassion. We experience wholeness. When we are able to hold compassion for ourselves and process the painful experiences we may carry, we can do the same for others. Our collective future, our personal healing and growth, are interwoven. As a being on this Earth, our lives do not take place in a vacuum. I do not believe it is a goal to rid ourselves of pain or discomfort, but instead to accept and tenderly process them into our wholeness, allowing us to see the wholeness in others. When we can alchemize our painful experiences into inspired action, that is where our collective power lies.

What we bury within us takes root and grows. What is buried within our lineages can manifest itself in our actions, our behaviors, our habitual patterns, and our mechanisms for coping. This could be said of the collective state of the world. The risk to remain right where we are in climate chaos and extraction is more painful and dangerous than the risk it will take to choose a different and unknown path of healing.

Today I stand on unceded **Sauk** and **Meskwaki, Hoocąk** (Ho-Chunk / Winnebago), and **Očhéthi Šakówiŋ** ancestral land. What does it mean to stand on land that is not yours? I surmised that Haiti, the tiny island nation of my mother's birth, would hold the key to all my unanswered questions. My mother immigrated to the United States when she was just seven years old. She didn't carry with her all the memories and knowledge I wanted to have. Am I still connected to that land? The tiny island nation where the native Tainos were slaughtered by the Spanish and enslaved populations were ripped from their homes in West Africa and forced to work on plantations in cruel and inhumane conditions. If anything, my answer lies in the resilience, strength, and fortitude of my shared blood. An island of enslaved Blacks rose up against the colonial powers as they had remembered their roots and their sovereignty and birthed their own liberation. What seeds of courage within me have been sown from birth? What can we learn from the wisdom in our bones about how to break free and birth new ways of being on this earth?

Often in the soil of our being, we have weeds, brambles growing in our garden that we did not plant ourselves. These inputs in our foundation affect how we grow. Having access to material resources, along with land, security, and stability all affects our ability to grow and prosper. What our ancestors experienced and lived through affects us in multitudes.

Collectively, our deepest wound lies in the root and in the earth. The earth star chakra represents the ground of all beings: the past, our collective consciousness, our ancestral lineages, and our relationship with the earth. Our connection with the earth, our ancestors, has been under siege for the last six hundred years, when Indigenous Europeans were forced off their commons; land was privatized; women's bodies were targeted; earth-based, animist religions were decimated by rising monotheistic religions; and imperialism and colonialism spread to every part of this Earth. I believe this is when our understanding of ourselves as creations of the earth, for the earth, and by the earth was fundamentally altered. Religions and spiritualities at this point worshipped the female body as the sacred embodiment of the creative fecundity of Earth. Humans lived by and worshipped the Earth and seasons; they were inherently interconnected.

How do we reclaim what has been taken from us? By remembering the old folkways and stolen earth-based practices, the loss of which has caused cultural and spiritual amnesia. Folk traditions, rituals, and earth-based practices cultivated a personal connection to earth and a sense of community beyond societal structures. We need to delight in the beauty and goodness of the earth and rediscover these practices. We need a swig of sweet elderflower tea while weeding the garden in the hot summer sun. This is our root work and where a new way begins.

Alienation, disillusionment, and disconnection are at the root of our mounting problems. Modern society can make us feel constricted and stuck. The natural world expands our vision and helps us remember our oneness. There is a reason Indigenous knowledge and lifeways are at the forefront of solutions for ecological repair. They have remained rooted, grounded in the reality of being on this Earth in reciprocity, guided not by ego but by the collective good. Most Western societies, capitalist and colonial-driven societies, remain untethered, floating in a virtual reality where identity and individuality feed our egos and insecurities. When food appears on shelves in supermarkets as if by magic and packages arrive on our doorsteps in a day, we obscure the true costs of labor, time, and energy. We are disconnected. How do we even begin?

I, too, straddle these worlds, one where convenience is king and easy, and the other a deep ache, a longing for something different, something more grounded. I know deep down someone, somewhere is paying the ultimate price of their body, their land, and their sovereignty for my convenience. There is an energetic thread that connects us all, like the mycelial network underground. Actions and intentions ripple out into our immediate relationships, our local environments, and the global field through commerce and connectivity.

Yet our compassion is contingent on who we view as kin. What if we understood the whole world is kin? How can we broaden our perspective to grasp the other as ourselves and the whole world as kin? Humanity is complex, multifaceted, not black and white. How can we embrace the shades in between that paint a whole picture instead of dwelling in binaries?

- The antidote to the overwhelm of this time is joy in communing with the plants.

- The antidote to hopelessness is carried on our breath.

- The antidote to the individualistic nature of capitalist white supremacy is community.

Singing to Our Bones, Listen for Their Call

It is my hope this book serves both as a field guide and a trusted companion. A sanctuary as you hold space for your loneliness and confusion, because I feel that way, too. I don't have all the answers, but what I've found as an antidote in uncertain and overwhelming times is to feel my emotions move through me like seasons, to share them with trusted hearts, to gift them space and time in my world, and to compost them and alchemize them with the earth. The earth is there to hold us and to create this existence. Connecting with the earth and seasons, I can continue to nurture myself, honor sacred time, and find joy in the little things, with the plants as my guide.

This book is an exploration of the plants I know and love and use in my day-to-day and an invitation into growing your own awareness, unleashing your creativity, and tending to your resilience in the Anthropocene. While I cover plants that are regionally available here in the Midwest of the United States, I tried to choose plants I thought would be more widely distributed. In our current society, we have instant access to a miscellany of choices, material goods, and information, all we could ever want. We are constantly researching, investigating, and probing to make the "best" choices. I hope this book is an invitation to see things in a slightly different way—to experience things for yourself and get your hands dirty.

Here we will cultivate kinship with the earth, grow our awareness of self, and experience the wisdom of the plants around us to form deeper, more meaningful relationships with them. Plants can become friends and allies in both good times and in times of hardship, and it is in relationship we dwell in hope.

We Are Connected

We are bearing witness to a time unlike any other. Our ancestors, our grandparents and great-grandparents, lived through wars, through famines, plagues, and political upheaval, but our human-made catastrophes are far from anything they faced. They did

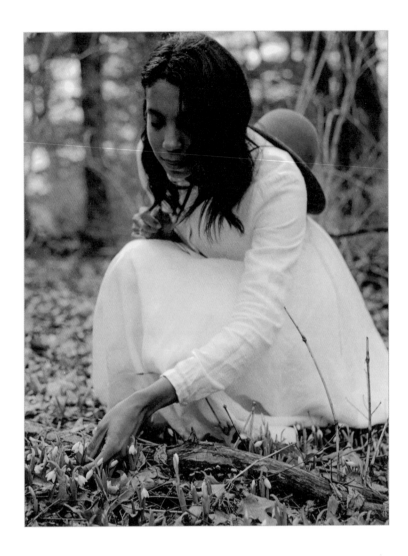

not have the level of awareness and information we have today, information about how our consumption affects the planet, about how chemicals affect our bodies, our waterways, and our planet. There seemed to be a veil of comfort and innocence about how those who came before us lived. And when we look back, there is a nostalgia deep in our hearts about the simplicity of their eras. But at the same time, there was deep inequality and oppression.

So how do we as people in the age of information and at the brink of climate disaster stand with eyes wide open and act accordingly? How do we respond to this moment? With courageous, healing hearts and open minds.

If I learned nothing else in my undergraduate education, it was that *we are all connected*. In both the little ways you would expect and in much greater ones. Emotionally, spiritually, physically, we are connected to those in our lives, the earth, our ancestors. The people who grow our food, the women who make our clothes in a factory halfway across the world. The family member we argue with, our children soaking up our guidance, the person across the country struggling to feed their family. What we do with that knowledge and understanding is vital to our survival on this Earth.

There is still time to limit climate change, IPCC experts suggest. Strong actions, regenerative practices rooted in Indigenous knowledge, preserving ecosystems that are carbon sinks, and sustained reductions in emissions of carbon dioxide (CO_2) and other greenhouse gases could quickly make air quality better, and global temperatures could stabilize in twenty to thirty years. We are already beginning to experience the chaos and catastrophe that is projected to become worse if we continue the way we have. We are not a carefree species that can live without consequences. Can this moment in time be a conduit of healing for us all?

As the climate crisis and ecological destruction intensifies, it is apparent that we cannot close off our hearts in the face of conflict and we cannot rely solely on our minds to solve the dilemmas we face. This time requires us to expand, to see beyond ourselves and to see beyond this moment to imagine how to face conflict and do repair work together. As we live through the unveiling of colonialism, patriarchy, and racism, I've come to understand my body is in a constant state of freeze, flight, stress. Enter the intersection of climate chaos and motherhood, and some days it feels too much to bear. And so, I turn to the plants in devotion, as I've come to understand our interconnectedness.

I've found plants not only have a unique ability to heal my intergenerational trauma and accumulated stress but are able to strengthen my stress response and resilience because of their unique sentience. Plants as teachers can help us process anger, grief, resentments, and soften our hardened hearts. Plants have played this role throughout our human story. Plants are food and tools for biophysical healing and spiritual guidance. The knowledge of herbalism and learning to listen intuitively to plants helps me feel prepared for the reality of climate uncertainty, and it is my hope this sacred relationship with plants can do the same for you.

Tuning into the seasons offers us information, opportunity to refine our healing and to connect with ourselves and the earth. When we live in alignment, we can cultivate ease and flow. In these pages I weave recipes, rituals, and seasonal rhythms to ease emotional distress, to provide nourishment, comfort, and a portal to healing.

PART ONE

A WOUNDED WORLD

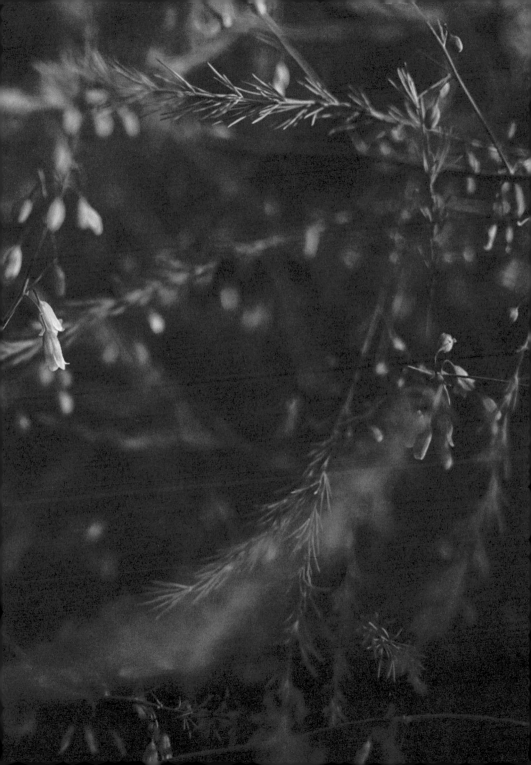

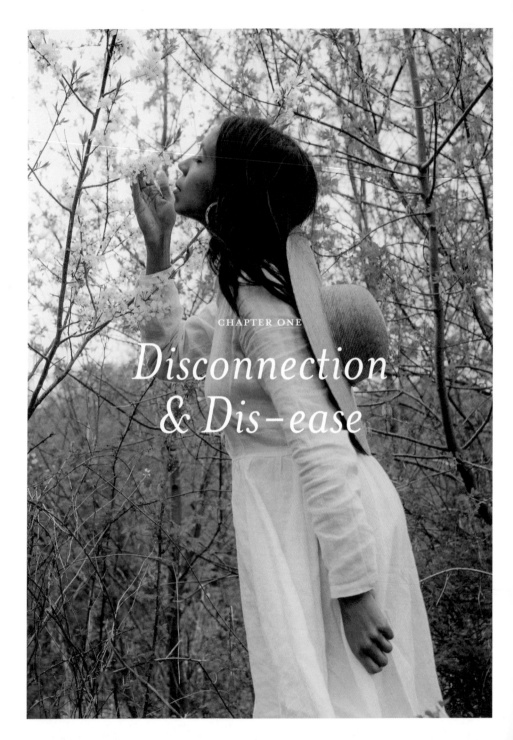

CHAPTER ONE

Disconnection & Dis–ease

"Pain is important: how we evade it,

how we succumb to it, how we deal with it,

how we transcend it."

AUDRE LORDE

When we are stuck, hurt, grieving, or healing, there is a plant that craves an intimate relationship with us. Plants inform every part of our human experience. Our food, our homes, the pages of our books, and our medicine all originated from plants, especially before the creation of synthetic materials. We are a part of the natural world. Prized goods in our modern societies—sugar, coffee, pharmaceuticals and drugs, electronics—are plant and mineral based. Our human-built world is dependent on the natural world, but our current relationship is an exploitative one. How can we come back into a relationship with the natural world to heal? We often look outside ourselves for grand, complex solutions and futuristic technologies to save us from our problems, but what if the solutions we seek are right under foot, buried in our ancient and imperfect human ways?

The body under capitalism is seen as a tool for labor and capital accumulation. For those with enslaved ancestors, that is a felt experience. Our bodies enslaved, our families destroyed for another's monetary gain. Under capitalism today, those roles are more diffuse, but there is an omnipresent concern with productivity. I find reclaiming my rest, my play, and my joy is a liberatory act. We have cultural amnesia about the other ways that humans have organized themselves and been in relationships with Earth, because at one point or another, those ways were demonized and devalued.

Today, facing a global pandemic, environmental collapse, and widespread anxiety, it is clear the ways in which we've been living are not sustainable. We have two options: to either adapt or die. Millions of human beings around the globe are already suffering from starvation, the climate crisis, genocide, and the pandemic. Extinction is a very real threat, yet we can't seem to stop, pivot, and change paths to heal ourselves. Our current systems and the exponential economic growth models don't have room for rest, for shifting course, for healing.

The proverbial clock is ticking on humanity. What can we learn from the natural world as we face human-made problems in both our internal and external worlds? Can we return to living with the earth and reclaim our spiritual connection and knowledge of plants? How can we slow down from the rush of the capitalist systems to create sacred space and ritual to do the intimate and vulnerable work of processing our grief, anxiety, and despair?

Healer and writer Prentis Hemphill reiterates that "our social systems shape our emotional landscapes and how we see ourselves in this world." Individually, we can map out our personal landscapes and understand the threads of our pasts to forge a way forward. We'll need to do this work universally as well. Wellness and resilience is for everyone. It shouldn't be complicated to value our own care and tend to each other. We all deserve *wholeness*, woven through daily rituals, rhythms, and routines.

How do we remake our world to be life-giving instead of destructive? Many of the world systems as we know them are built on domination. Earth's systems evolve from relationships and reciprocity.

Domination Systems

What are the psychological and physiological effects of racism, discrimination, and poverty? What are the effects of the demands for perfection and unwavering indifference of bureaucracies in the face of pain and trauma? What beliefs are reproduced in our social and religious systems?

According to systems scientist and author Riane Eisler, in the domination model and societies, there are "in-groups" and "out-groups." Humans are socialized and hardwired to be kind to the in-group for survival, and a consequence is that individuals in the out-group are labeled inferior and dangerous. Eisler's belief is that humans have an enormous capacity for caring. In domination societies, difference in form (e.g., male or female) is equated with superior versus inferior. We internalize it for gender, race, and so on, and it keeps us from establishing a relationship. We've learned to dominate the "other," pushing away instead of holding a spirit of curiosity. When I learned to hold disparate parts within me, opposing pieces and multiplicities, I found great healing. How can we learn to embrace difference and cultivate a spirit of curiosity about the diversity that makes life so rich? Diversity is a value we need to hold close to our hearts as we navigate the challenges facing humanity.

Living within systems of domination means we have cut off parts of ourselves to stay safe. The domination and extraction we see on the macro scale is happening on the micro scale in our bodies and our relationships. We carry these experiences either firsthand or through intergenerational trauma, wherein the trauma is passed down through children and grandchildren. We now know, through a growing field of research called epigenetics, that experiences of hardship and trauma can leave their mark on future generations.

In my own personal experience, the first step to processing trauma is a calm nervous system and a safe space. A trauma is a problem until it is processed. We must be willing to integrate our trauma. When our trauma is unhealed, we can project it onto others and enact violence in our words, thoughts, and actions toward others. Plants can help us feel safe enough to understand the ways in which we dominate ourselves and each other, and instead gain a sense of compassion for the shared experience of humanity. Doing this work can help us feel more whole.

In our current model of extraction and domination, when you are looking for roots you will take from others. But we can develop cultural practices to acknowledge and process traumas, grief, anxiety, old and new with the plants as our guides. As a Black woman, I grew up trying to please other people, thinking that was where my safety lay. My trauma became my standard operating procedure, a constant state of stress in my body.

I understood this response to trauma as a part of my personality and not a safety mechanism, until I reclaimed and befriended my own thoughts, inklings, needs, desires, and boundaries. I'm unlearning, rebuilding my foundation from my roots up, remembering how to put my relationship with myself first. This process of reclaiming self is important to our work healing the earth.

Our actions, our decisions ripple throughout the web of life. If we hold that fact in our awareness, can we let that guide our actions? Can we stop and consider whether we are on autopilot, re-creating storylines from the past?

By healing our personal wounds, we can respond to the needs of the present moment rather than perpetuating our traumas on each other and the earth. From my personal experience and the everlasting journey of personal healing, I see a glimmer of hope. To enact real change, we must be willing to imagine. To take care of each other. To come back, again and again, to the possibility of change. Because if we don't, we will perish. By examining different ways of living, new ways of being with ourselves, each other, and the earth, we can nourish rather than dominate.

Ecological Disruption

For the past few years, the intensity of climate events has unfolded before our eyes: flash flooding, tornados, extreme heat, drought, severe thunderstorms. Some nights, I watch our beloved apple tree through the blinds thrash in the wind, a parade of thunder and lightning illuminating it. As heavy rain pelts our steel roof, alarm rises in my belly. I'm awestruck, reminded of the sheer power of nature and how much is out of our control. Climate chaos is here, taking on various forms, but we cannot look away.

There is a growing body of evidence that suggests deforestation due to land development and industrial agriculture is giving rise to diseases. Not only does deforestation cause ecological and biodiversity loss (and the rapid release of carbon, which contributes to global warming) but it also increases the spread of animal- and insect-borne pathogens. Due to complex interactions, deforestation gives rise to infectious zoonotic diseases, such as malaria and dengue fever. As forest habitats are destroyed, animal populations and human populations come closer together; with the destruction of habitat, wildlife makes homes near our homes, increasing the likelihood of disease spreading between the populations. Protecting nature protects us as well.

This is a climate emergency as well as human rights, public health, and ecological emergencies. As we destroy old growth and rain forests, they release stored carbon into the atmosphere. We destroy habitat for wildlife and often push out and displace Indigenous populations. Deforestation, fires, and droughts decimate biodiversity and create global health risks. Dwindling water resources spark civil wars, grabs for finite oil resources fuel wars, inequities caused by development and emerging global markets over local ones, rising seawater as a result of melting polar caps are leaving island nations uninhabitable, and devastating rainfall and floods contrast with droughts and wildfires. Plants are also suffering from habitat loss, overconsumption, climate change, and fire suppression. Many native plants need our conscious effort and ability to develop ecological awareness. Wherever you are on this Earth right now, climate chaos and extreme and unpredictable weather events are becoming more and more common. But we cannot *normalize* them, because there is nothing normal about it. Now is the time to fortify ourselves and find solutions in each other and the earth.

"Ours is not the task of fixing the entire world at once, but of stretching out to mend the part of the world that is within our reach."

CLARISSA PINKOLA ESTÉS

The Kindred Nature of All Sentient Beings Is Real and Alive, if We Listen

Plants are complex, highly evolved beings that have lived for millennia, and they continue to evolve, adapt, and change depending on their environments. We are still learning about the sentience and reciprocity of plants. Trees communicate with each other by sending carbon, sugars, and nutrients through their roots. A mother tree will send nutrients to younger trees through the mycelial network. Mycelia not only produce the fruiting bodies known as mushrooms, but they form dense, expansive responsive networks woven into the soil of forests and in our garden beds to assist the plants. Mycelia mine the soil to make nutrients more bioavailable to plants, and plants send carbon down their roots into the mycelia to be stored in the soil and feed organisms in the soil. Flowers attract bees to pollinate and feed them. There are so many wondrous life-giving models of relationships and lessons held within the natural world. The earth and its rhythms speak of deep time, and the natural world works in patterns, cycles, and reciprocity. In order to learn how to slow down, to be patient, and to be resilient for whatever happens next, we must pay attention. Many problems in our human-built world feel dire, but the healing I've found on the plant's path is one of support, hope, relationship, depth, and the ability to change.

We assume that we cannot change, because the problems that exist are so much larger than us. Change is out of our control, but it is also inevitable and a natural part of life. But we individuals make up the system. Our individual experiences and pain are not singular, and neither are the solutions. If the living world has anything to teach us, it is a message of interconnection and constant change, of reciprocity, responsiveness, and adaptation. A large part of what is missing from our relationship with the earth today is our ability or willingness to listen deeply and make changes based on the information we receive, to make our systems flexible, our borders malleable and adaptable to the necessary changes. When we as individuals are wounded, it affects the whole living system.

How do we heal? How do we remain flexible and responsive? Our complex problems cannot be solved with simplistic answers but require a metanoia of our homes, our hearts, and our relationships to ourselves and the world around us. This transformation is made easier in connections and relationships with the plant world and each other. Plants offer a portal. Over time, when we grow them in our gardens, when we prepare them in a tea or eat them in a meal, they offer their innate wisdom and healing. They nourish us, heal us with their biochemical properties, and, with their energetics, they can help shift our awareness and remind us of our interconnectedness.

What we do, how we live, how we act affects other beings and ripples throughout the web of life. When we are acting from a wounded place within ourselves, it affects the people around us. We are truly not individual actors; we are part of the organism of Earth. Nurturing that awareness may be the only way to sustain life on this planet. In comprehending our interwoven nature, our actions must be all encompassing

The silver lining to that interconnectedness is interdependence. When we heal, it ripples outward. When we act out of love, it changes us and others. We can each cultivate an intentional and intuitive relationship with the earth and the plants for healing our wounds—physical, spiritual, and emotional.

When we can tune in to our local environments and the ecosystems around us, we are more capable of becoming advocates and voices for change and environmental protection. The belief that we humans are separate from nature is one of our greatest human fallacies. If we can humble ourselves, ask for help, and slow down enough to listen, plants can guide us in embracing the uncertainty of this new age, much like they held our ancestors in dark times. Plants can teach us how to remain flexible and open to what the present moment has to offer. A tree with deep roots can weather many storms. Plants can be battered by the wind yet right themselves. Plants not only can help us process our grief and heal our bodies, but they can help us build our capacity to act instead of reacting to what lies ahead. They can help us attend to the biochemical nature of chronic stress in our bloodstreams.

In my experience with plants, from a simple tea to time spent with my hands in the dirt, there are ways to build capacity, to remain flexible, and to find connection in trying times. When our containers grow larger, we can process, heal, and grow.

The earth cannot heal without our hard work. We must clear out the old from our hearts and minds to envision the new, and our intentional input is necessary. We must comprehend that the fundamental disconnection of our human societies from the earth, its cycles, and its wisdom has harmed us all. In this book, I share everyday ways to connect to the earth around you for resilience, resistance, liberation, and collective healing. Restoring kinship and connection is essential to saving our planet and healing ourselves.

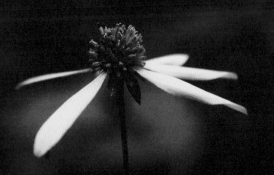

CHAPTER TWO

Ecological Grief & Anxiety in the Anthropocene

*"Shame corrodes the very part of us
that believes we are capable of change."*

BRENÉ BROWN

O ur ecosystems are being quickly and fundamentally altered. Humans have experienced ecological grief over time, from having an old tree in your neighborhood cut down or losing land to suburban development, needing to migrate because a water source disappeared, to beloved animal species going extinct. There are losses, seen and unseen but felt by the collective.

While you may not be experiencing this where you live, this is the current reality for many. As environmentalist Vandana Shiva uncovers in her writing and work, "Those least responsible for climate change are worst affected by it." Former colonized countries and dispossessed peoples are experiencing the burden of extreme climate events. In Ghana, the combination of neocolonial development and urban planning and extreme rainfall has left thousands displaced and revealed their human vulnerability. Ancestral trauma is familiar to them.

Climate change is posing a threat to all aspects of human health, from mental health to physical well-being, through extreme weather events and natural disasters and the trauma and stress impacts of those. Generally, insecurity due to climate change is causing acute and chronic stress conditions because of forced migration, food insecurity, floods, and changes to landscapes. The mental health conditions resulting from global climate change are rooted in ecological anxiety, uncertainty, despair, and hopelessness.

Communities already vulnerable due to social, racial, and economic inequalities will be the least resilient in the face of climate chaos.

Folks across the world are experiencing ecological grief as their landscapes are changing. Even those who aren't as directly affected by climate change experience ecological anxiety and hopelessness that our future, our existence, is so uncertain. How does that really feel? I feel ashamed, hopeless, and powerless in the face of it all. Where do we start?

Shame

Shame is a painful emotion; it causes humiliation or distress. It is another collective condition that can hinder our growth and ability to change the way we behave.

Humans are destroying our home. Our daily actions and ways of being exacerbate the conditions, yet we can't seem to escape them. Our hands are tied by the system in which we all exist. I am not immune. I must drive a car to get to the store to feed my family, although I know driving is bad for the environment. I must fly to see my family. I cannot afford a hybrid car. I cannot afford living in the most sustainable ways. We cannot buy our way out. Capitalism would have us believe that if we buy a certain wooden dish brush

and stop using sponges, our guilt will be scrubbed away, but this diverts our attention from the real issues at hand and the major players at fault.

There are alternative means of living, but because we don't live in a "free market," there is very little access to those alternatives that can help change our ways and reduce harm to the planet. Thus, we feel shame. Shame as an emotional response narrows our perspectives, keeps us in our ego, and limits our ability to connect and see beyond. We can overcome shame through acknowledgment and compassion for self. There are also specific plants I turn to, to support self-worth and self-love.

Breaking Down Grief

Grief is a necessary yet painful part of the journey in accepting that a part of our life has changed. We are experiencing a collective grief—the ways in which we live and what we value need to shift and change to support the planet. We are confronted with the effects of our daily behaviors, habits, and relationships. We are grieving a changing landscape, the loss of natural habitats, and consequently watching plants and animals suffer. When someone dies, there is a collective and socially acceptable ritual for processing this grief and loss. With climate chaos, ecological changes, contamination of our water-

ways, destruction of forests, and species extinction, there are few socially acceptable or collective rituals to process this pain and loss.

How can we collectively ground and examine this in a way that helps transform the grief from helplessness to empowered action? How can we normalize our suffering, normalize sharing our experiences, create rituals around integrating painful emotional states, and allow healing to happen? Firstly, by understanding and moving through each stage of grief.

What Is Grief?

Grief is deep sorrow in response to any kind of loss. It can be an overwhelming, all-encompassing, and incredibly strong emotion. Grief has physical, cognitive, behavioral, social, cultural, spiritual, and philosophical dimensions. It is an embodied experience that can lead to depression and anxiety as well as physical symptoms, such as heart problems, decrease in immune response, digestive issues, body aches and pains, sleep disturbances, and unhealthy coping mechanisms. The mind, body, and spirit are not separate elements.

Of the twelve interconnected systems in the human body, the immune, cardiovascular, digestive, and nervous systems are most susceptible to the effects of grief. Increased blood pressure, chest pains, irregular heartbeats, and heart attacks are all physical symptoms associated with the biochemical stress grief can have on the cardiovascular system. Grief is extreme stress; it can lead to gastrointestinal issues as well as aches and pains, shortness of breath, anxiety, headaches, fatigue, heaviness in the body, and muscle weakness. It can also cause neurological issues including confusion, decreased attention span, memory loss, headaches, and brain fog. Humanity has experienced a global pandemic, and we're facing our Earth being destroyed. It has both physical and emotional effects on our bodies. But is the root of this grief and its effects being recognized as such?

When it comes to shame, grief, trauma, and other emotions that we've been conditioned to bury, they are often not a collective experience. I believe living through the Anthropocene, climate chaos, and the global pandemic is an opportunity to embrace the very real pain we experience, connect in vulnerability, and navigate the uncertainty we are faced with as an opportunity for collective healing.

What We Bury Takes Root in Our Lives

Grieving ritual: We all carry heaviness and pain from experiences and losses. The heart and the lungs are connected, the heart expressed in the hands and through the voice. Grief is held in the heart and expressed through the throat chakra. Scream aloud, silently, or into a pillow so that the universe can hear your pain and acknowledge it. Once you've released it from your body, you can weep, cry, and reclaim sovereignty over your being again.

There are five states of grief: denial, anger, bargaining, depression, and acceptance. These are descriptive states—not prescriptive. Grief is not linear; rather this terminology gives us a framework to understand our emotional responses to our rapidly shifting and changing world. The states of grief originally mapped out by Swiss American psychiatrist Elisabeth Kübler-Ross in her book *On Death and Dying* are not absolute, but I do think they describe a range of emotions that humans are experiencing as we face the reality and consequences of our systems.

Depression

Conditions on our planet are destabilizing. It can feel uneasy, and you may feel at a loss as to what to do at times. You may feel the weight of the world on your shoulders but do not know how to make a difference. It often manifests, for me, as feeling stuck. Depression is characterized by sadness and a loss of interest in things that once sparked joy. Depression can be biological, the lack of as well as too much of certain chemicals in the brain, but it can also be triggered by an uptick of cortisol due to stressful life events.

Depression can both inhibit the brain's ability to function and affect attention span, memory, and our ability to plan and make decisions. It is a common disorder and a growing experience for many in the face of ecological disaster, racial inequalities, and climate inaction. For me, I find this happens when things I once loved no longer seem important in context with these larger global happenings, and as I begin to unravel how capitalism has affected people and the land for centuries, I become overwhelmed. As a woman of color, these wounds run deep.

Denial

Denial is seen as a rejection of basic facts and concepts, even though there is scientific or social consensus because it is psychologically uncomfortable. It's a natural part of the healing process to experience denial, but it may cause people to blame others, suppress their emotions, and rationalize the problem instead of working through the conflict. Denial can arise out of our very human desire for emotional security. It can be caused by anxiety and fear; to cope, we deny our experiences and the experiences of others instead of dealing with the root emotions.

We've all experienced varying degrees of these feelings, but what comes with them is repressed emotions that deeply affect psychological well-being. Denying our feelings leads to cognitive dissonance, which can cause damage to ourselves and those around us. The only way out is through.

Anger

Anger, I admit, has been an uncomfortable emotion for me to own and process; I often feared I'd be misconstrued as a hostile Black female for expressing my displeasure and my deep upset. Yet as I began to befriend my anger, I realized it gave me a burning clarity and signified things that were ultimately very important to me.

Anger is defined as a strong feeling of annoyance or displeasure. I found anger to be a strong motivator to use my voice. Anger can be a secondary emotion we shift into when we are actually feeling fear, loss, and sadness; a way of regaining personal control when feeling those more vulnerable emotions is to shift into a state of anger. In traditional Chinese medicine (TCM), anger is said to affect the liver, and the emotional imbalance can cause physical issues, and vice versa.

I know I experience a sense of rage

when I hear from the United Nations that we have twelve years to avoid climate catastrophe and yet nothing of substance is done. I feel a sense of hopelessness and anger that someone must be held accountable. Anger rises within me in the face of injustice, but anger can also swallow all other possibilities. Anger can be blinding. Anger is an emotion that I have been afraid of for most of my life. In my healing journey, I've learned anger, like other emotions, is a language of our bodies, alerting us to imbalances. In terms of climate change and social injustice, we need to find a way to channel the energy of our anger into action. We can use our anger to motivate and fuel intentional action, like the heat rising in bellies and our hearts, to show us what we value and then pour it out to create changes in our community.

Bargaining

This is an inability to accept reality. You attempt to delay your emotional process and the reality of your feelings: "If I do x, y, and z, it might alleviate the consequences and the pain." You might even believe trading one thing for another will change the outcome.

Acceptance

Acceptance is a place of healing, the beginning of receiving and embracing what is without resistance. Acceptance allows us to let things flow in and out without attaching, without judgment, and without denial. How can we move through the parts of life that are uncomfortable, accept the emotions we are experiencing and the reality of our lives so we can move forward with creativity, grace, and peace?

Resistance to natural emotions causes further pain. Acceptance does not mean we like, want, or are choosing something, but it can give space for ease, and even a sense of peace and happiness. It is from a place of acceptance we can confront reality with a clear mind. In working with plants, I've found the capacity to sit with my own emotional experiences and the experiences of others. Making a cup of chamomile tea helped me confront childhood shame. Lemon balm in the winter shakes off the mental fog of depression and rekindles the light of joy in the darkest months of the year. In relationship to plants, healing at all levels of our being unfurls.

Ecological Anxiety

Anxiety can cause our bodies to enter a state of flight or fight, releasing stress hormones. Our systems of domination and oppression cause our bodies to be in constant states of anxiety. Our parasympathetic nervous system never gets the chance to put our bodies into a state of rest if we are always worried what is going to happen next.

Ecological anxiety is fear and worry about what will happen in the future, worry about what decisions should or

Herbs for Anxiety & Ecological Grief

Bee Balm (Monarda fistulosa)

Hawthorn (Crataegus *spp.*)

Holy basil, tulsi (Ocimum sanctum)

Lemon balm (Melissa officinalis)

Linden (Tilia europea)

Multiflora rose (Rosa multiflora)

Reishi mushroom (Ganderma lucidium)

Rose (Rosa *spp.*)

Thyme (Thymus vulgaris)

Violet (Viola *spp.*)

should not be made in the face of un-certainty and unforeseen events. And with climate chaos, we are experiencing a heightened sense of fear of the unknown, uncertainty of what the future holds, and that registers as a deep underlying sense of dis-ease in our bodies. The first time I felt ecological anxiety, I was rocking a four-month-old Magnolia to sleep for her nap. I was gazing into her eyes as she drifted into deep comfort, and I began to experi-ence a discomfort rising in my belly. What should have been a joyful moment shifted into dread as I tried desperately to think about who she might be at fifteen. I had a sudden realization that our world will look very different in ten or fifteen years' time if we do not act in potent and meaningful ways today. Our children may not know the general ease and stability we grew up with. Ecological anxiety is keeping many people from having families because of the unknown, and the uncertainty of our ecological landscapes.

Environmental philosopher Glenn Albrecht coined the modern term *solastal-gia*: "the distress that is produced by en-vironmental change impacting on people while they are directly connected to their home environment." This concept em-bodies the powerlessness and the lack of control over the unfolding process of eco-logical change.

We should be alarmed, but if we are operating out of urgency, out of a state of collapse, freeze, or shutdown, it lim-its our ability to see clearly and to create connection. Chronic stress and sleepless nights can elevate cortisol in our bod-ies, diminishing our immune function and leading to burnout. With the ability to regulate our nervous system through nervine plants, we can be more flexible in our response. If we can tap into a state of aliveness—a deep and abiding aware-ness that our time here on earth is finite, everything here is sacred, this place is the heaven we seek, and in this moment lives the potential for creativity and inspira-tion for a new vision—we could work on enacting change instead of being afraid. Embracing the depth of pain and radical joy is the key to our wholeness and clarity of vision.

The earth can ground us and teach us about right relationships. Our emotions, like the plants, are our teachers and can be guides.

Our human species has evolved deep relationships with plants, and they are available to us at any time to offer deep healing. Plants are powerful because they work on the subtlest levels of our energetic and physical bodies to make big shifts in our awareness and consciousness. Plants can help us cope.

CHAPTER THREE

Sacred Earth, Body & Home

When we move through this world with intention and act with purpose, we can shift energy in our bodies. Our bodies are intimately intertwined with the earth and each other. There are four layers of an individual: the physical body, the emotional body, the mental body, and the spiritual body. These layers interact with each other and can be either in balance or out of balance. This energy also interacts with the world around us, influencing others. The plants can help balance these different layers of our energy. There are also interplay and feedback loops between the layers, which is why a physical ailment can affect our mental and emotional outlook or a mental illness can cause pain within our bodies.

How can we make a practice of honoring our emotions as teachers? Think about when you feel grief. What hurts? When you experience depression, where does it linger? When you are overwhelmed, where does it land? Where do these states exist in our bodies? When you have anxiety, do you get a stomachache? I do. The roots of energetics lie in many ancient systems that have come to inform Western herbalism. Ayurveda is a traditional, ancient Hindu system of medicine and healing based on balancing body systems by working with energetics. Traditional Chinese medicine similarly works with balancing the elements within for healing. The chakra system, which arose out of ancient Indian sacred texts known as the Vedas, is one way to interpret information. Chakras are interpreted as wheels or cycles of energy located throughout the body. They inform where trauma, emotional pain, self-doubt, or overwhelm goes in the body and how it connects to our psychological states. From there we can understand what plants we can build relationships with to help us with the work. Modern science has shown the classical seven chakra centers contain high concentrations of nerves intersecting with the spinal cord.

What are you holding and where? Linguistically, our language holds idioms to discuss this deep connection between emotional states and the body, such as "butterflies in my stomach" to discuss anxiety, "weight on my shoulders" to relay feeling a burden is too much to bear, "stabbed in the back" to explain betrayal and heartache.

Our physical bodies process, absorb, and store repressed emotions, energies, and experiences that can result in physical ailments and illness when we do not do the work to heal, process, and work with our trauma. Our body receives, processes, and integrates internal and external stimuli through our nervous system. Our nervous system consists of three main parts: the central nervous system, the peripheral nervous system, and the enteric nervous system. The central nervous system receives messages from other parts of the body and interprets and controls the responses. The peripheral nervous system is connected to the organs, which send messages and information to the central nervous system, the brain, and spinal cord via the peripheral nervous system. They all work in tandem.

The organ systems correlate with emotional states by way of our nervous system. The peripheral nervous system is made up of the autonomic nervous system and the somatic nervous system. The autonomic nervous system is split into the parasympathetic nervous system and sympathetic. The peripheral nervous system responds to external stimuli through our senses of touch, taste, vision, smell, and hearing. It controls breathing and heartbeat. This sends messages to our brain, which interprets the signals and reactions. In the central nervous system, how we think or interpret the stimuli dictates how we respond or react.

Our sympathetic nervous system works with the endocrine system, which oversees hormonal output to control our fight-or-flight responses. Our heartbeats quicken, our breathing becomes shallow—this is our immediate response to dangerous situations so we can react in a way to keep us safe. If our day-to-day lives feel unsafe and we are in a constant state of stress, vigilance, or hyperawareness, our nervous system, our hearts, our blood pressure, and our bodies are affected. Symptoms of an overactive sympathetic nervous system include increased heart rate, elevated blood pressure, anxiety, fatigue, and insomnia. It can make us feel drained and exhausted, leading to adrenal fatigue.

Our parasympathetic system is the system of "rest and digest." It is activated when we feel safe and calm, and when we are asleep, and it helps our bodies recuperate. Activating the parasympathetic brings the body back into balance. It helps repair and restore our nervous system. It helps us move from a state of anxiety into calm. Plants can also help us get to that place. Slow, deep belly breathing, somatic practices such as yoga and stretching, massage, spending time in nature, engaging your senses through touching your lips can all activate the parasympathetic system and help our brain learn to cope.

Traditional healing modalities have not siloed the human experience, and their approaches to wellness see the human body as a whole. These modalities consider how our environments and imbalances can lead to illness. According to traditional Chinese medicine, the heart center and the lungs hold grief; our kidneys and bladder, located near the solar plexus, hold our sense of fear and powerlessness; our stomach, spleen, and pancreas carry our anxieties and insecurities, like lack of trust or control or when things are hard to digest. The liver and gallbladder, the detoxification system of our body, process our anger and frustration. Liver stagnation sees mood swings and low energy. Our reproductive system, our sacral chakra, and our sexual organs, or root chakra, hold issues surrounding insecurity, childhood, and family trauma. We can hold either excess emotion or deficient emotion in these organ systems, which results in different symptoms.

As plants have their own properties and energetics, we might find we are called to certain plants because they are sympathetic to what is going on in our own bodies. Plant intelligence can work on the systems of our body, thus releasing the blocked emotions.

Embodying Our Healing

The World Health Organization (WHO) defines health as a "state of complete physical, emotional, mental and social well-being and not merely the absence of disease" (Grad, 2002).

The human nervous system is a vast network throughout our body that controls its functions. Our movements, our breath, our digestion, the sensations in our bodies, our thoughts are all connected to this system.

My background as a practitioner of yoga and registered yoga instructor introduced me to the chakra system, and it has become an important lens in my toolkit for understanding my body and healing. Ancient codified and earth-based systems of medicine and healing, such as Ayurveda and traditional Chinese medicine, along with Indigenous practices developed and refined over thousands of years, work in the realms of balancing the body-mind-spirit connection to achieve states of healing. Yoga is more than physical asanas; it is about self-reflection, bringing the body and mind into communion.

Western medicine and psychology are beginning to catch on to the knowledge that we cannot compartmentalize ourselves. I do not use chakras as a means of bypassing physical illness. I have found it helpful to understand my healing not only from a biomedical standpoint, utilizing modern medicine, pharmaceuticals, and therapy, but seeing a broader picture of health as it connects to a wider spiritual, emotional interplay. We can utilize a variety of modalities to gain perspective on our complex internal ecosystems.

Sometimes physical pain and other emotional, mental, dis-ease, dis-comfort are the body's indicators of problems within the system, influenced by outside systems like the environment, family, relationships, and culture. Western allopathic medicine does not often look at the whole person: it does not take into account diet, family history, socioeconomic background, trauma history, social life, and mental and emotional life, yet it prescribes pharmaceuticals targeted to one specific ailment, because it sees the symptoms as the problem, not as signposts pointing to the root of systemic imbalances.

Capitalism instills urgency and has us living in constant states of nervous system dysregulation. I think about nervous system dysregulation like a small baby who doesn't know how to calm itself. If all their material needs are met, a mother or caregiver can pick up a baby, lay the child against their beating heart, and sway like the waves in an ocean, and the baby will be soothed. In doing so, heartbeats sync, nervous sys-

tems match, and the caregiver grounds the baby's energy. When I step onto a yoga mat or into the woods or my garden, I plug into a wider experience of myself and the world around me. Grounded, soothed, I am lulled into state of calm.

I've run away from my feelings because they felt too big for me to hold or understand. But there is a powerful moment when we let our physical senses, actions, emotional body, and subtle energy coexist—an alchemy of healing when we are present with the reality of our existence.

If we can take the time to listen to our bodies, to accept our experiences, we can heal ourselves and unlock our innate and somatic wisdom. We can listen more closely to the stories our bodies tell, as our primary home.

The Earth Star

The earth star chakra is our human connection to Earth. An energy point located twelve inches below our feet, it is our personal, energetic link to the earth itself. From where life springs and where it returns, the earth star holds the spirit of the bones, the rocks, the interconnectedness with our ancestors, the soil from which all life arises, our collective consciousness, and our own personal energetic connection with the earth beneath our feet. It is where our roots are planted and fed. I named my herbal apothecary for this chakra, because at the time I was turning to the flowers to illuminate deep-seated intergenerational patterns, beliefs, and

traumas. It is the soil beneath our feet, the bones of our ancestors and the life force that connects us all. I work primarily with flower essences; flowers are the highest expression of a plant that grows from the depths of the soil, carrying a message of healing for us on its petals. Working with the earth star chakra can help us understand the nature of all life. The earth star chakra is the beginning and ending of all things, reminding us that earth provides everything we need and connects us all.

When we work with this chakra it serves as an anchor, helping us cultivate a sense of stability, increasing our awareness of interconnection with this earth and all other life. No matter the issue at hand, life and death will continue; while our culture fears death, it is necessary, inevitable, and nourishes what life comes next. What habits and patterns can we turn into fertilizer for living?

Root (Our Foundation) — to Have

The root chakra, muladhara, located at the base of our spine, is our foundation. Its physical correspondences are with the lower sexual reproductive system, the rectum, tailbone, legs and feet, and blood. Physical manifestations of imbalances in this chakra include disorders of the bowel and large intestine, ailments of the bones and teeth, eating disorders, and issues with legs, feet, and the base of the spine, all of which can manifest as frequent illness.

We can conceptualize the chakras as places throughout the body where the nervous system convenes. What thoughts and experiences tend to cause blockages in this space in our body? Events such as unmet bodily needs, malnourishment, abandonment, sexual or inherited traumas, poor bonding with parents, or issues with survival can manifest as low energy and a lack of vitality. An imbalance or blockage in the root chakra can mean we have a fear of change and suffer depression. I experience this when my anemia flares up. Anemia is an iron deficiency, a literal deficiency in my root chakra, the blood, the building block of the body. Physically, the circulation in my body is low, I lack energy, I feel cold often. These physical symptoms can also manifest as depression. When I am able to get my energy up through nourishing foods, nettle infusions, and iron sup-

plements, the fog from my mind begins to lift, and I begin to feel like myself again.

This chakra is concerned with grounding, nourishment, trust, home, and health. It is about the roots of our being, our family systems, and our childhoods. In a balanced state, we assert our right to be here. We challenge systems of hierarchy and work to cultivate safe spaces for Black and brown bodies in our communities.

Traditionally, the root chakra can be balanced by reconnecting to our body with movement and safe touch, grounding with the earth and eating root vegetables, such as beets, carrots, and sweet potatoes, and nutritive herbs with a high mineral content, like nettle, purslane, dandelion root, and burdock root. Feeling ungrounded and craving security can manifest through a desire for and consumption of material objects to help us feel safe, which creates a false sense of security. Instead, make a cup of nutritive nettle tea. Nourish yourself before going into a situation lacking. Spend time feeling your feet on the ground and reaffirm that you deserve to take up space. Your ancestors carried you this far and you are valuable because you are alive.

PLANTS TO WORK WITH: Roots, including beets, burdock root, dandelion root, nettle.

Sacral (Our Inner Waters) — Emotion

Women go to the waters to bathe, to bring back drinking water and water for cooking; they share their hardships at the water and find themselves anew. Running water brings new life and washes away old skins. The waters need to be protected and they, in return, bring life. The inner waters are where our life begins in the womb, giving birth to creation.

Our sacral chakra is located in our lower abdomen. Called svadhishthana in Sanskrit, which translates as "where the self is established" and can also mean "sweetness," this chakra involves pleasure in the simplest form. It is the root of the sexual organs, the place in our body that holds the ability for creation in its physical and spiritual forms. Our sacral area in the most physical sense is connected to where our spleen, reproductive organs, urinary tract, uterus, and kidneys are housed in our bodies. Sensuality, sexuality, desire, and reproduction rule our emotional waters and needs. As a Black woman, I grew up afraid of my own sexuality and my creative powers, afraid of drawing too much attention, and it felt unsafe to truly embody the seat of my creative powers and potential. I worked with flower essences, hibiscus, and plants like damiana to process what lived in my hips. Dancing and movement spilled stories of sexual abuse in my family lineage living within me. I had to come to terms with the notion that it felt safer for me and the women in my lineage to dull their powers than to have full expression. As women, our bodies are valued for the beings we produce, but that is the extent of it. We are controlled and shamed for being overly emotional or sexual, leading to a blockage of our creative life force energy. This leads us to not being able to trust ourselves and the life force flowing through us.

When doing the emotional work connected with this part of our body, it is the mental and emotional world of boundaries, trust, emotional attachment, warmth, and intimacy. What do we do when we do not feel "enough"? We are insatiable, there is a hunger and desire for more. Nothing is truly enough, but an antidote is self-love and pleasure. Traumas and experiences that affect this chakra are sexual abuse, emotional abuse, enmeshment, manipulation, alcoholism, denial of feelings, sexual desires, and needs. An imbalance in this chakra leads to overconsumption of all things to fill a void.

This chakra is associated with physical disorders of the reproductive organs, painful menstruation, urinary tract system, adrenals, blood sugar, sexual dysfunction, frigidity, low back pain and knee trouble, deadened sense, and a loss of appetite for pleasures in life. We can find healing in this chakra through movement, dance, emotional release, and boundary work.

PLANTS TO WORK WITH: Hibiscus, raspberry leaf, yarrow, rose.

Solar Plexus (Our Inner Fire) — Our Will Power

The solar plexus, manipura, is located in our gut right near the navel. It is a place of transformation, where we convert food into nourishment, where we digest information and create power to fuel our bodies. This energy center connects with our pancreas, stomach, liver, and small intestine, as well as digestion and mental energy. The physical manifestations of the imbalances and blockages in this energy center include eating disorders; digestive disorders; chronic fatigue; disorders of the stomach, gallbladder, pancreas, and liver; and diabetes. There is also a lesser known part of our body's nervous system located in our gut, called the enteric nervous system. The enteric nervous system's network of nerves, neurons, and neurotransmitters extends along the entire digestive tract.

Because the enteric nervous system relies on the same type of neurons and neurotransmitters that are found in the central nervous system, some medical experts call it our "second brain." This second brain in our gut, in communication with the brain in our head, plays a key role in certain diseases in our bodies and in our overall mental health. Because of the brain-gut axis, gut problems can cause anxiety, and anxiety can cause gut problems.

The solar plexus chakra is the seat of our ego identity. It is where we transform our will into action and establish control over self and others, beliefs, details, and constructive versus self-critical thoughts. With a healthy balance, it is from this chakra we can learn discernment and cultivate intuition, trusting your gut but not acting out of ego. Mental imbalances include perfectionism and shame. A balanced solar plexus chakra allows one to embody warmth, confidence, spontaneity, responsibility, and personal power. Traumas and experiences that lead to imbalances in the chakra include shaming, authoritarianism, domination, physical abuse, fear of punishment or retaliation, and oppression (including racism and patriarchy). To confront white supremacy, you must be willing to sit with your own entitlement. For a Black or brown or Indigenous person, confronting white supremacy within means accepting your inherent worth and value, seeing all of the ways and behaviors you've acted out of a sense of low self-worth. Over- and under-inflated sense of self is the work of the solar plexus.

PLANTS TO WORK WITH: Herbs that support our personal power, self-esteem, and fire. For low self-esteem, seek out solar flowers, like calendula, that warm our digestive fires. Calendula can help you listen to yourself, while fennel, mint, chamomile, and St. John's wort work on our relationship to identity and how we use our energy in the world. Bitters help us digest and rest.

Heart (Our Shared Air) — Love

The heart chakra or energy center is connected to the thymus, heart, lungs, circulatory system, blood pressure, lymphatic systems, and immune system. The Sanskrit name, anahata, translates to "unstruck."

The heart pumps blood throughout the body. Our hearts never stop beating, and our lungs never stop breathing. They work in tandem. We breathe, respire, to bring oxygen from the outside world into our blood. Our blood carries oxygen to nourish our tissues. When our heart races, out of anxiety or panic, deep belly breaths soothe us. A heart needs support. In TCM, the heart holds an energy and a spirit called shen, which is nourished by our blood. When our blood is not flowing well and there is tightness and constriction around our heart space, it can leave other parts of our body susceptible to illness. We can feel numb to the world, and it may be harder to give and receive energy in the form of love. Our emotional hearts can also affect our body. When heartbroken, we can feel sluggish. How do we process our grief and open our hearts to love and new possibilities? Our hearts are our centers: we create, love, and connect from our hearts.

Physical ailments connected to this system include respiratory allergies, heart problems, circulation and immune system disorders, breast issues, and asthma. Traumas associated with this chakra include rejection, betrayal, abandonment, constant criticism, and unacknowledged grief. Wounds to this chakra can manifest as tension between the shoulder blades and pain in the chest. The emotional and psychological effects of a blocked or out-of-balance heart chakra include jealousy, coldness, withdrawal, loneliness, depression, and self-sacrifice.

A balanced heart chakra lends itself to harmony, compassion for others and self, intimacy, trust, ability to give and receive freely, openness to new ideas, and growth.

PLANTS TO WORK WITH: Rose, hawthorn, lemon balm, thyme, and violet, among others. Blood-building herbs and nervines help support our hearts to feel nourished and safe.

Throat (Sound) — Purification

The throat chakra, vishuddha, represents open and clear communications, resonance, self-expression, thoughts, creativity, speaking up, listening, releasing, breathing, and the life force. The physical manifestations of imbalances, overstimulation, and trauma related to this chakra include illnesses of the throat, thyroid, parathyroid, neck, ears, respiratory system, sinuses, tightness of the jaw, and speech issues. Vishuddha translates to "purification" and what it means to use your voice as an expression of self and how that is clearing and purifying.

As a Black woman, I learned at a young age to bite my tongue. But I can still remember my first protest in college—I felt alive chanting in unison with others; we were a flock of geese synchronized, loud and marching together. Feelings from deep down in my body were channeled through my throat chakra and given wings. When expressed, our feelings make ripples of healing through our bodies. Sharing our heavy truths gives them places to live outside of our bodies, and we can mold them into beauty and sorrowful creations.

This chakra can be healed through storytelling, ancestral practices of oral traditions, humming, singing, and making art, as our hands are seen as extensions of the throat chakra. The throat chakra is the portal for the expression of the lower chakras. Through writing and self-expression, along with talk therapy, we learn how to communicate and when it is appropriate to choose silence. Emotional imbalances of this chakra include too much talking, poor listening, secrets, and gossiping. Humming, like the sounds of the bees and the vibrations of the world's heartbeat, is used in healing practices of shamanism and chanting.

Traumas with the chakra are connected to lies, receiving mixed messages, constant yelling, criticism that blocks creative expression, and threats. My absolute favorite ritual for my throat chakra and a pinnacle of expression is throwing my head back, opening the throat, and howling my grievances and gratitude at the full moon. Howling is an act of purification under the rays of the silvery moon.

PLANTS TO WORK WITH: Throat-soothing sage; demulcent plants such as mullein and marshmallow to help our words slip out.

Brow (Light)—to Perceive

Sometimes I need to close my eyes to truly see. When I've taken in too much information and sensory inputs—my children banging blocks, my to-do list running through my head as my husband is singing, music playing in the background—my nervous system is overloaded. I learned a handy trick from my yoga training: rub your hands together until some warmth is created and place them over your eyes. Calm washes over, if only for a moment. Our third eye chakra, ajna, represents our ability to see clearly. Our central nervous systems process outside stimuli for internal information. This chakra affects our ability to interpret and translate information.

This energy center is centered around our minds: our ability to imagine, visualize, and dream, where self-reflection and perspective happen. It is from here we can make choices for the good of all in service to the community and be a witness to the activity of lower chakras.

Traumas connected to the brow energy center include invalidation of intuition, technology and information overwhelm, frightening environments, war zones, and environmental degradation. Imbalances and physical manifestations of trauma in this energy center include poor memory, lack of imagination, obsessions, and nightmares. Trauma can reorganize the mind and change how we think (Van Der Kolk, 2014), but our neural plasticity means that, with help, we can think new thoughts and create new pathways.

PLANTS TO WORK WITH: Lavender allows our nervous system to regulate and rest so we can have clarity and calm, rosemary facilitates blood flow and helps us remember ourselves, and nasturtium flower essence also helps ground buzzy energy in the mind into the body.

There is overlap between the brow and crown chakras, the functions and capacity of the mind. There is a shift between brow and crown that has to do with a greater sense of collective awareness, the former having the function of taking in information while the latter holds the beliefs that organize our information.

Crown (Thought)—Our Collective Consciousness

The crown center is where our ability to perceive, analyze information, and build thoughtful understanding occurs. It informs our ability to be open-minded, to question, and to connect with a spiritual understanding and greater wisdom. The "thousand-petaled," or sahasrara, chakra focuses on our ability to relate to the wider world and a greater sense of consciousness.

In yoga or meditation, something inside me will shift for a moment, and I perceive my higher self, witnessing the chatter in my brain. This is the ability to see a thought for what it is but not attach to it. This chakra is connected to the pineal gland, the central nervous system, and, more symbolically, the head and the hair. I think of bathing or baptism; it is here our spirit is cleansed and born anew. We can ritualize washing our hair, cleansing unwanted thoughts, and open our channel to more positive ways of thinking and clarity.

It is from this place we cultivate compassion, oneness, empathy, understanding, and a sense of a higher power.

Traumatic experiences that affect this chakra include misinformation, forced dogma, invalidation of one's beliefs, blind obedience, lies, learning difficulties, and excess in the lower chakras. The physical manifestations can include cognitive and mental delusion, confusion, amnesia, and migraines. When we can connect to our higher self and to a greater spirit, we can be guided out of ego states to have a universal understanding and greater compassion for others. Imagination gifts the opportunity to envision new possibilities. Without imagination, there is no hope, no change to envision a better future, no place to go.

PLANTS TO WORK WITH: Lavender, reishi mushrooms, tulsi (holy basil).

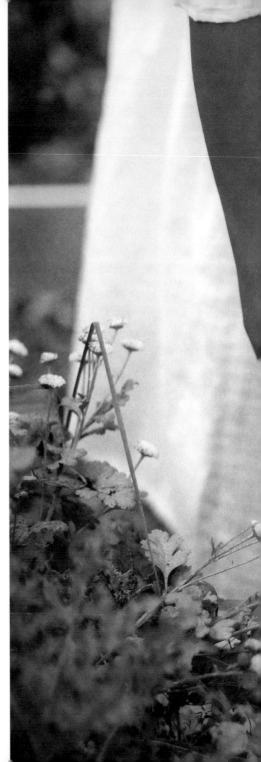

There are more than 114 chakras connected to hormones, neurotransmitters, and glands. The chakras are an ancient and esoteric way for humans to conceptualize themselves as whole energetic organisms, where physical ailments, spiritual expression, and outside influences interplay.

These are all tools enabling us to understand the nexus of physical, energetic, spiritual, emotional, and psychological to heal ourselves and, in turn, reconnect with the Earth. We cannot outthink our dis-ease, our disconnection, but through the often uncomfortable and typically hard work of embodiment and connection through the earth, we can heal. Embodiment is not about clearing the mind to achieve some altered, elevated state of reality, but to be rooted firmly in the present moment. The chakra system indicative of our nervous system acts as internal markers, the outward expression of imbalances pointing to where our locus of personal and interpersonal healing work needs to be done.

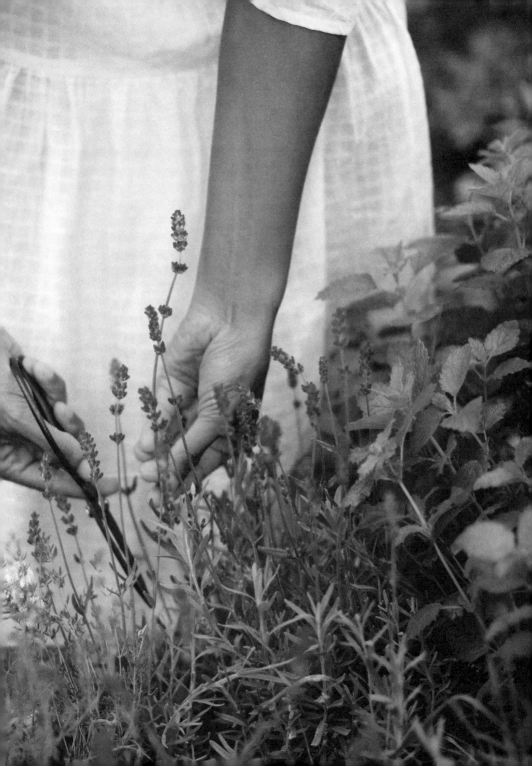

PART TWO

Intuitive Herbalism

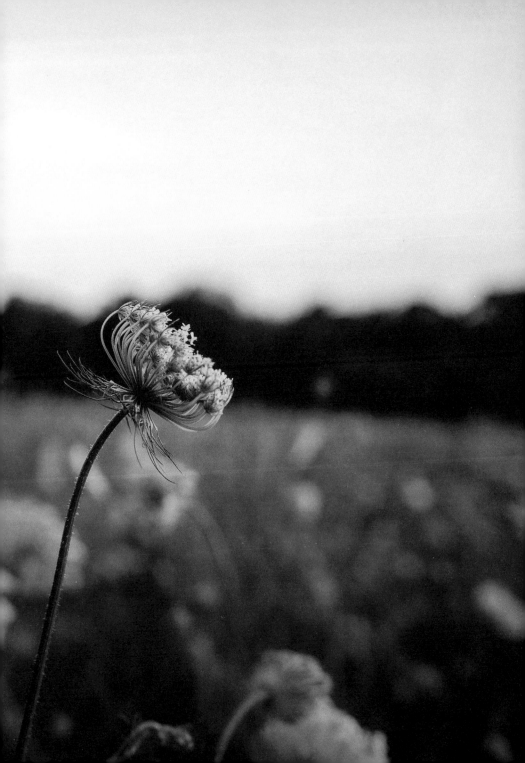

CHAPTER FOUR

Human Kinship with Plants

We belong to the land; the earth does not belong to any one of us. Every being, human and nonhuman, on this earth is kin. And this is our beloved home.

Our connection to the earth, to the plants, to the stars and the moon is our birthright. Humans once were given the gift of knowledge passed down to us through our traditions, our cultures, our elders. Today we may need to dig a little deeper in ourselves to uncover our natural connection to the earth, its species, and to understand our place here. Six hundred years of capitalism and colonialism have uprooted us. Many of us were dislocated from our homelands, often by force, and made to fit into prescribed boxes and ways of being unlike what we had ever known: slavery, Indigenous genocide, and schools to break folks of their connection to their native language, culture, foods, and sense of self and identity. Hierarchies were drawn with white men on top, with people of other cultures and the land, its resources, and animals below them.

Not too many generations ago, maybe your grandmother's grandmother, or even your own grandparents relied on their direct connection with the earth for sustenance, to grow their food, make their clothing, and build their shelter. My great-grandmother Nan grew food from her garden for her fourteen children and her wider community. She relied on the earth for survival. In pagan religions,

people prayed to gods for rain and for prosperous harvests. It wasn't a passing fad—the earth, its cycles, and its resources were the most vital relationships we had as humans. Today, with globalization, we are less aware of the ways the earth is our lifeline; it is less immediate in our lives. We see this relationship reflected in the dollar sign at the market or on the news, but many people in Western societies are insulated from the fragility of our existence and our inherent dependency on the earth for survival. However, it's becoming harder and harder to ignore that relationship.

My personal connection to plants really began with a desire to understand and demystify these connections. To cultivate integrity between my values and my lifestyle. Consider a simple box of strawberries on the market shelf. What does it mean that a farm worker in California's Central Valley grows the strawberries? Are they conventional or organic? If conventional, because they are the more affordable option, is the farmland sprayed with endocrine-disrupting chemicals and are the farm workers exposed to them? Does the agricultural runoff with pesticides and petrochemicals flow into the local water sources? Do bees come to feed off the nectar of the strawberry blossoms in spring? Have they brought those persistent and bioaccumulating chemicals back to the hive? Is that now in the honey I stir into my tea? If the answer is yes to this series of questions, in what meaningful ways can I divest from these systems? What is the actual energy and input it takes to grow the food that sustains my life? How can I do less harm, if possible? I started to purchase organics when I could on a college budget, purchasing from local farmers' markets, but I became intrigued: Could I grow my own strawberries? What inputs, labor, time, land, and knowledge would that take?

In following my thread of curiosity, slowly unraveling and unveiling the web of capitalism that ensnares me, I became interested in what plants grew around me and their uses. That thread led me from my cherished California nature in search of a slower pace in the Midwest. The possibility of owning a home for the first time in my life without overworking. Maybe we could garden and grow some of our own food and ascertain what it takes to sustain ourselves.

When my husband and I moved our family from the city to rural Wisconsin, we purchased a house from a local herbalist. The garden she established would begin to answer some of these questions for me and open my story to so many more. Less than an acre, the soil she worked, nourished, and tended to create a mini ecosystem in town would help me understand the deeper threads and questions about connection, nourishment, and reciprocity. As I was knee-deep in early mothering, I was re-mothering myself in the soil of the garden and the language of the plants. I engaged in experiential learning about our roots and our kindred relationship to plants.

Our abiding connections to the moon, the stars, the seasons, the plants, and the planets guide us. Many Indigenous traditions and world spiritualities recognize this truth and that all living things carry messages of abiding truth. When we can work with the elements within us and connect with the elements outside of us, it can bring our lives into balance and we can cultivate a sense of harmony and ease, even in the face of great conflict and growing uncertainty.

A Place of Solace

As I've done research to learn more about how my enslaved ancestors worked with plants, I've come across narratives and anecdotes suggesting many enslaved Africans on plantations in America relied on a direct connection with plants. They were familiar with plants from their native lands, often their knowledge of farming practices and plants being the reason they were targeted for agricultural work in the colonies. Through living and working and trying to survive, they had exposure and relationships with various Indigenous peoples, incorporating that knowledge of the plants as well as relying on intuition and their senses to learn what plants to use and for what. The woodlands, swamps, and meadows were a haven from enslaved life on plantations, and the plants were friends, teachers, and healers. They crafted and filled out their diets and medicine cabinets with plants found and foraged. With what meager means given by their oppressors while their labor and lives were capitalized and exploited, they made the most of the environment and connections around them to survive and thrive. This connection provided not only physical sustenance and healing of ailments but a transcendent spiritual connection with a foreign land.

Shortly after the system of slavery was ended, the system of oppression continued in the creation of laws that made it illegal for former slaves to "trespass and forage." What was once used as a balm was outlawed, and our roots to this act of resistance and reverence became forgotten. Today we can reclaim our sovereignty and sense of belonging in the forest, woods, and wild. It is imperative to return land to Indigenous communities and help Black communities reclaim relationships with the lands that have been systematically taken away. I grew up with a fear of the wild, a fear of the unknown and getting lost in the woods. Now I know these wild places are portals to return to the root of our humanity. Foraging is an act of resistance.

I haven't come to know all the plants of my disparate ancestors, the native plants of their lands and how they used them, but I have the gift to connect with the plants on the land where I stand. Here I root, I acknowledge, and I endeavor in my flawed humanity to be a steward of the earth. Beginning a relationship with the bioregional herbs, plants, and ecosystems in your immediate environment puts you in direct communication and kinship with the earth. Observation is the first step to devotion. In *Working the Roots*, Michele Lee preserves the stories and reclaims the traditions of African American herbalists firsthand. Counter to today's culture of overconsumption, elders would use only a handful of herbs, making good friends and establishing relationships with a few solid plant allies. Our grannies, our elders, our midwives, took to the gardens and the woods to find the good weeds to help those in need.

I often wonder what plants my great-grandmothers, on both sides of my lineage, turned to in times of need. Did she use yarrow or plantain to tend to a scraped knee or make an infusion to help settle an upset stomach? What plants did she know by heart? I've wondered about my ancestral connections with plants, but there is no such record in my family. Because knowledge was passed down from mother to daughter or female relatives, what happens when this thread is frayed?

Hopefully this book mends a gap in generational knowledge, an ode to the forgotten wisdom and a guidebook to leave for my children so they know the good weeds. When we work with whole plants, they in turn work on many layers

Ritual

This is an exercise to connect with one plant that has been calling to you this season. Whether on a hike or a walk through your neighborhood, you can use this ritual to connect with a plant.

Find a quiet and safe place to sit. Settle into your body. Observe your natural breath. If you feel safe, close your eyes. Inhale and at the top of the inhale, pause and exhale, lengthening the time of the exhale. Do this for a round of six breaths. When you are done, open your eyes, hold the intention to find a plant to connect with. Walk slowly and maintain an open awareness. Take notice of a plant. Is it swaying in the wind? Might it be calling you into connection? If so, come closer. Observe its color, its structure. Gaze at the plant. Do you feel a resonance with this plant? If not, move on to the next plant. Practice this ritual with open awareness a couple times before you identify your plant. Ask permission to take a cutting and bring it home with you.

Identify and learn about its uses. Do any of its healing properties resonate with you?

of healing: physical, emotional, psychological. Plants are synergistic. They work on body systems and beyond. A plant that works for one person may not work for another, which is why it is important to understand our own bodies and the energetics of plants. But it is equally as important to understand that the breadth of how plants work is beyond just our scientific understanding. Many Indigenous societies and religions revere plants as sacred. Let us rekindle this type of relationship with plants beyond the scientific knowledge and identification tools. Not only to alleviate wounds and help us achieve states of wellness, but to build relationships and to allow us humans to become more responsive and adapt with the ecosystems around us.

What if we could identify more plants around us? What if, in building relationships with the forest and fields, we could know what was ailing them and how we could help? What if we didn't see a tree just as a resource to be consumed, but an elder?—A being that has stood in one place for hundreds of years witnessing various changes and life-forms moving in and out of its perceptions.

Before we can confidently embark on our exploration, we need tools and vocabulary for a firm foundation. There are many ways to work with plants, and there are about 390,900 species of plants out in this world. There is emerging research that shows plants have a consciousness and intelligence networks akin to our own. Plants exist on different timescales than humans, but plant energy or consciousness can work with our own.

It's important to understand we don't need to know all the plants. As a child, I believed that I needed to be friends with everyone. My mother reassured me that a few good friends would do just fine, and those few friends might also change over time, depending on the season in your life. Let us find a few good plant allies to invite into our hearts and homes, season by season.

Intuitive Connection to Plants

At the first herbal conference, I attended a workshop about direct connection with plants. The teacher introduced the concept of the doctrine of signatures, a methodology to learn and ascertain information about plants. The doctrine of signatures dates from the fifteenth century and states that herbs resembling various parts of the body can be used by herbalists to treat ailments of those body parts. A plant gives us clues as to how it can be used for humans through its similarities in its structures, color, smells, shapes, textures, and the habitat it grows in. This workshop started with a meditation, because when we clear our minds, we have an ability to pick up on cues and listen more deeply. Then we went on a hike. Like I said, this was my first conference, and I didn't know half of the plants we were visiting in this forest, but I correctly "guessed" or intuited the plants' usage from direct connection and deep listening to plants.

One example of this happened after I returned home. I spotted a flower I had never seen before blooming in the prairie garden in our yard. It was pink and erect, with lots of tiny blooms and familiar ribbed leaves. My daughter Magnolia and I were sitting at the dining table, and she spotted it out the window and said, "Mommy, that looks like a heart." The blooms indeed were heart-shaped. Later I found out that the plant of the rose family was called *Filipendula rubra*, or queen of the prairie, and was indicated for heart issues. What I learned in this workshop was that the plants have many ways of communicating with us.

Plants come to me when I need them most or when someone in my life needs them. There is a resonance between a person and the plant. There is even evidence to suggest this was one way our ancestors began to interact with plants—through trial and error, but also through an intuitive connection.

This connection can be cultivated by anyone to help them bond in a deep and meaningful way with the plants around them. This section will outline the tools and means to begin. Once you start tuning in to the plants, herbs, and flowers around you, you'll start seeing them everywhere. Is there a plant following you around? A plant, a tree, a flower from your childhood or memory that stands out? Are you having a hard day, are you depressed or anxious, what plants do you notice around you? What are their herbal

RESPONSIBLE & ETHICAL FORAGING & LAND STEWARDSHIP

Land Acknowledgment Ritual

I acknowledge the Indigenous lives, sacred practices, and tribes of the land I stand on as a way to honor their knowledge and existence. Diversity of thought and language is one of our greatest tools of resistance against homogeneity. Indigenous peoples and their practices are interwoven with the land and all of its inhabitants. I challenge you to find out what peoples are indigenous to the land you live on and explore why they are no longer there.

Find a patch of grass, a bench, or a quiet place to ground. Sit quietly on the earth. Inhale the air shared by us all. Imagine your sit bones rooting into the earth. Open your heart and mind to the people before you who inhabited the land you sit on. Imagine a time without concrete buildings, subdivisions, and paved roads. A time when the sun and moon were timekeepers, the creek was the water source, and the soil gave life. In this moment, get curious about what relationships might have felt like for those living at this time. What plants were growing? How did the landscape differ? Acknowledge the value of different ways of seeing, the way time flows, and different means of knowing. Take a moment to acknowledge the pain, the stories of loss, oppression, and suffering the land holds.

actions? Find resonance with the plants calling to you.

As Robin Wall Kimmerer shares, our awareness is key: "Our indigenous herbalists say to pay attention when plants come to you; they're bringing you something you need to learn." Herbalists often talk about this occurring for a population or ecosystem, that an abundance of a plant will arise in an area that needs that plant's particular healing power. The same can be said of the seasonality of plants. For example, dandelion leaves come up in the spring for clearing and detoxifying the system after a long winter's stagnation. Elderflowers blossom in the summer months for cooling us on hot days and elecampane roots are harvested in the fall for respiratory health in the winter months ahead.

We can all connect with plants in our everyday lives. Simple preparations make it easy to build a relationship with plants and find a sustainable source for healing and nourishment. I found working with one plant at a time, learning its form, its name, and its song became a portal for personal healing and those around me.

You don't need all the herbs; a working relationship with just a few will change your being. When we cultivate a direct connection with the plants in our ecosystem, we weave new traditions and deeper interdependence. In learning about plant medicine, I also want to acknowledge the cultural appropriation and lack of recognition of the lineages which the medicine we are using comes from. This does not mean we cannot participate in and learn from these lineages, but it's important to acknowledge the history of colonization that has occurred around the world. We can learn where the plants originated and the names Indigenous people know plants by, not just the Latin nomenclature. We can learn about Indigenous peoples' relationships with the plants to help deepen the context in which we use plants. These foundational practices rooted in decolonizing the natural world can impart context and meaning in other parts of our lives.

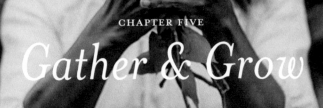

CHAPTER FIVE

Gather & Grow

*I*n this chapter, I outline tools for everyday herbalism. I outline simple preparations, tools, and a basic vocabulary to begin to familiarize yourself with herbal knowledge, both scientific and intuitive.

I was so nervous to begin using plants, partly out of fear that I would hurt or even poison someone. It's a valid fear, as caution and awareness are important tools in our toolkit and should be exercised when entering relationships with plants. But I think in the process of slowing down, using our senses, listening to our intuition, and growing our knowledge of the ecosystems around us, using a few good plants in your everyday life can be incredibly powerful and transformative.

Observation

Observation is an action of devotion, a beautiful instrument to connect with the world around you. Commit yourself to wholly seeing. Slow down, tune in to your senses and commit your attention to another phenomenon outside of yourself. Gaze into the flame of a candle, or watch the clouds pass by in a state of equanimity and curiosity. I spent my first summer in our cottage garden observing the plants. Noticing the details of plants helped me begin to recognize them, not only as individuals but across the garden and our wider landscape. Plants travel and migrate; some grow individually or in stands. Plants that I first observed in the garden, I ended up noticing in parks, on the sidewalk growing between the cracks, on our drives. Observation takes time and leads to confidence with identification.

Identification

A teacher once told me there are over forty plant characteristics that you can find: leaf shape, flower structure, stem shape, hairs or no hairs, petal number, color, ridges, serration, and so on. Take time to identify the plant, forgetting the immediacy of our culture. Imagine you are courting the plant. Bring a field guide for your specific bioregion. Pay attention and be prepared to make mistakes. Get to know its likes and dislikes. Where is the plant growing? Observe; visit a plant a couple times. What keeps calling you back? What is its name? Correctly identify your new plant friend before deciding to work with it. After correctly identifying but before you harvest, take a minuscule bite of its leaf for its energetics. It took me a couple months of identifying plants in the wild and in my garden before I felt comfortable using them. Asking friends and fellow plant lovers questions about the plants builds community. Tending to relationships takes time, and cultivating a relationship with plants is no different. Bring a friend who is familiar with plants. That is one reason why I like growing a plant in my garden: it ensures I know what I'm using and harvesting and builds my confidence and connection with a plant without a shadow of a doubt!

Plant Characteristics to Look For

- **FLOWERS:** Count the sepals, the petals, and the stamens. Does the flower occur in a node or terminate at the end of the stem?

- **LEAF:** Is the leaf structure simple (a single leaf), compound (separated into distinct leaflets), smooth, or serrated? What is the shape of the leaf? They may be oblong, heart-shaped, very thin, and so on. What are the color and the texture of the leaf?

- **LEAF ARRANGEMENT:** How are the leaves organized on the stem? Alternate or opposite?

- **VEIN PATTERNS:** Are the veins parallel? Do they form a network (reticulate)? Are they paired on opposite sides (pinnate)?

- In what **SOIL CONDITION** does the plant grow?

- **WHAT SHAPE IS THE STEM?** Round or square? Are there hairs or thorns? Is it hollow?

- **DESCRIBE THE ROOT SYSTEM.** Does it have a taproot or shallow root system?

Foraging: A Practice in Reciprocity and Mindfulness

If you do not have access to space for a garden, and even if you do, I greatly encourage you to forage. Getting out into wild spaces is a deeply nourishing practice; befriend local and bioregional plants and realize how many plants exist around you.

While you may not have access to all the plants I discuss later in the book, I have no doubt you will discover equally powerful remedies and allies, as well as plants I have yet to meet. Before you decide to harvest, it is important to identify and be sure you are ready to process or use the herb you want to gather to make sure they don't go to waste. Walk by four separate groups of plants before gathering from the fifth stand you find to ensure there are enough individuals in that community to survive. Say a prayer of thanks to the plant, sing a song, bring an offering. This is a sacred collection. Approach the plants in a spirit of fellowship rather than thinking of a plant as a resource that is yours to take and own. You can find local places like parks to forage, or make friends with local or regional organic farms to see if they want your help weeding. Take your time getting to know your area and bioregion.

Plant Families

Once I began to learn about plant identification and plant families, a whole new world opened to me. I could see likeness across species, the interconnectedness, and I grew more confident in my plant identification and understanding herbal actions across families. Plants belong to a family, yet they take on many roles, actions, and forms; they don't just do or belong to one thing, and that is their strength. In knowing plant families, you notice similarities between plants, their seedlings, and their habitats. Plants within a family often have similar uses, patterns, and tastes. If you can begin to identify characteristics of the plant families, you will have a better understanding of what is safe and edible and how other plants may look similar at first glance but are not.

Alliaceae

The members of the onion family are biennial or perennial monocot plants growing from a bulb or corm. The leaves are flat and round and smell of garlic or onion when crushed. There are about 600 species, including chives, shallots, garlic, leek, and onion.

Apiaceae

With over 3,700 species in the carrot, celery, or parsley family, this group is identified by its compound umbel, hollow flower stalks, and taproot. Members of this family include carrot, angelica, dill, cilantro, and Queen Anne's lace.

Asteraceae

Asteraceae is quite a large family with over 23,000 species and has subfamilies. Dandelions, daisies, sunflowers, calendula, elecampane, goldenrod, echinacea, burdock, and chamomile are all part of the Asteraceae, or aster, family, as is yarrow. A key identifier of members of the aster family is a composite flower head made up of small disk flowers attached to a center disk. Think about how a dandelion head is multiple seed heads of spent ray florets attached to a center. This family has a long history in traditional medicine and provides medicinal and food plants like lettuce, chamomile, and wormwood.

Brassicaceae

This family contains more food crops than medicinal plants, but its inclusion helps demonstrate the likeness or kinship within a plant family. The brassicas of the mustard family include cabbage, broccoli, cauliflowers, kale, dame's rocket, and radish. The flowers of Brassicaceae family members have four petals, four sepals, and six stamens.

Lamiaceae

The Lamiaceae or mint family contains some of the beloved garden herbs—marjoram, peppermint, sage, oregano, basil, lavender, and rosemary—and they are cultivated for their culinary and medicinal uses. Lamiaceae includes over 7,000 species that are characterized by their square stems, opposite leaves, and aromatic and "mouthy" flowers.

Malvaceae

A few well-known and well-loved plants of the mallow family are the hollyhocks that dot cottage gardens, cotton, marshmallow, and hibiscus, one of the ancestral Haitian plants I've connected with. Worldwide, this family features 1,500 species, and is known for its mucilaginous and demulcent qualities, excellent for inflamed conditions like sunburns and sore throats. Mallow greens and flowers can be used. Mallow family plants have palmate, alternate leaves with funnel-shaped flowers with five petals and three to five sepals. Basswood and cacao are now considered subfamilies of the mallow family, which includes linden (*Tilia* spp.).

Rosaceae

This is one of the most beloved plant families, gifting humankind with fragrant flowers and delectable, often succulent fruit crops. The rose family includes roses, apples, peaches, pears, blackberries, raspberries, and strawberries as well as meadowsweet and hawthorn. They are commonly identified by their five-petal flowers with a cluster of many stamens in the center.

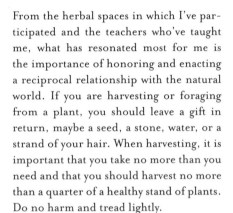

From the herbal spaces in which I've participated and the teachers who've taught me, what has resonated most for me is the importance of honoring and enacting a reciprocal relationship with the natural world. If you are harvesting or foraging from a plant, you should leave a gift in return, maybe a seed, a stone, water, or a strand of your hair. When harvesting, it is important that you take no more than you need and that you should harvest no more than a quarter of a healthy stand of plants. Do no harm and tread lightly.

Make a connection with a plant and ask for permission before harvesting to initiate a relationship. It is also essential that you have positively identified a plant

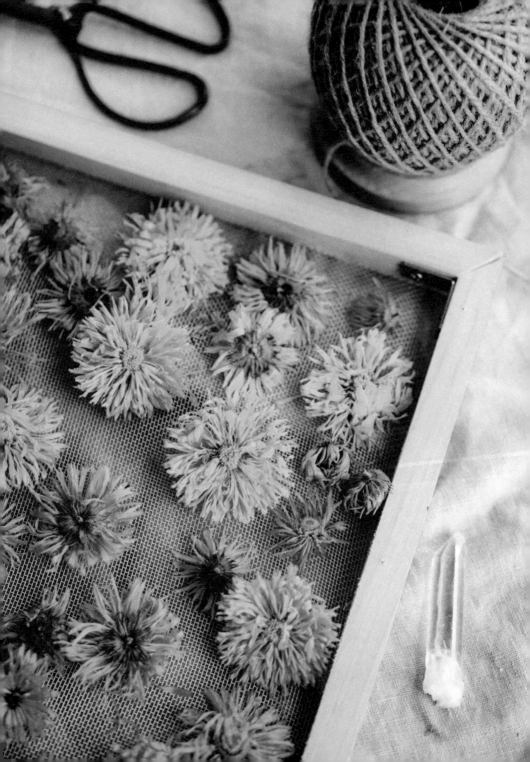

using this book or a comprehensive field guide before harvesting. Be mindful of where you are harvesting—at least a good one hundred feet away from roads, highways, and sprayed agricultural fields to make sure that the plant you are harvesting has not bioaccumulated the pollution, toxins, or chemicals. Now, what do you do once you've harvested your plant?

Harvesting, Drying, and Storing Herbs

When harvesting and drying herbs, it is important to harvest at the correct time of the season and stage of the plant life for each specific plant, and for the specific remedy you're using the plant for. There is a general rule: harvest bark and leaves in spring; bloom, blossom, and fruit in the summer; and roots in the fall, when the plant focuses its energy and life force into that particular system. You do not want to harvest endangered or at-risk plants, or take too much from a plant. Harvesting in the correct season for each plant increases its potency and ensures you are using the plant in the correct way.

In the spring, the energy of the plant is going into the leaves. They are more succulent and milder in the spring. In the summer, the energy of the plant is rising up to produce a bloom, if the plant flowers. It's a perfect time to harvest chamomile, calendula, elderflowers, and wild rose, while the bloom is fresh and at its peak. If you are looking to harvest roots from plants like dandelion, elecampane, and root vegetables, you want the energy previously sent to the leaves and flowers back down into the root.

Plants have multiple uses and edible parts. For instance, you can pick dandelion leaves in the spring for pesto, flowers to infuse in vinegar and tea in the summer, and the root for bitters and tea in the fall. The time of day is also important: harvest leaves and blooms in the morning after the dew has dried. Harvesting in the heat of the middle of the day can leave your plants dull. To dry leaves, stems, and aerial parts of a plant for storage, harvest by cutting them with a sharp pair of scissors or shears, strip the leaves from the main stem, making sure the leaf is green and well-shaped, and discard any leaf that has been bitten by insects or withered. You can dry stems, too. Spread them out evenly on a drying rack or screen in a warm place with good air circulation until they are brittle. Roots should be chopped fresh, while they are still pliable, and they often need more time to dry.

Alternatively, you can hang small bunches of herbs by string, lay them out on screens, or use a dehydrator on a low setting. When moisture has left your plants and they are crispy to the touch and crumble, you know they are ready to store. If they are not adequately dry, they will mold when stored. I store my dried herbs in jars, labeled with the plants' name and date of harvest, and out of the sunlight to preserve their medicinal potency. Dried herbs can last for a year, but check herbs for mold or moisture before use. Dried herbs should retain their smell and color; if they are looking lackluster, return them to the earth and compost them.

While ordering herbs online is a good option if you do not have access to growing spaces, working with plants that are bioregional and local is one way to connect with your community. Rather than creating a large carbon footprint trying to get herbs from other places or countries, seek out local farmers and purveyors. Find what plants grow around you and start from there.

Cultivating a Garden for Resilience

Gardens were our ancestors' way of hedging their resilience. Foraging seeds, season after season of cultivating strands of their favorite grains, fruits, and greens found in the wild. A way to root and create stability for their food sources. Our gardens have always been spaces and places to plant seeds of hope and determination. A place of growing food we know will sustain and nurture us. In the future, could small gardens, community gardens, and localized sources of food replace industrialized agriculture that depletes soil and contributes so much pollution? Should the role of growing our food go from the hands of the few to the hands and work of the many?

Victory gardens were planted during World War II as a buffer against food insecurity. Beyond that, gardens are a way to food sovereignty. There were summers where we were living paycheck to paycheck, with not enough income to go grocery shopping, so I made meals out of what was growing in our garden. In food deserts, where fresh produce on a market shelf is rare, gardens can be an alternative way to mitigate food insecurity. We saw a wave of new gardens planted at the onset of 2020 as a portal to healing and a tangible means of hope, creating a sense of security and sovereignty in times that felt out of control. Research suggests that the bacteria in soil helps our coping response to stress. Time spent in our gardens allows us to digest our personal and collective struggles while reminding us of the constant change cycles of life that ebb and flow. The garden offers us a place where we can take part in the natural rhythms of our Earth. Planting seeds gives way to new life, tending to and caring for a life and watching it grow. We harvest the fruit or flower or leaf, the physical manifestations of our love and energy, to nourish our bodies and share with others, and then we experience grief when the season ends. Our gardens provide us with the ability to see the cumulative effects of our diligence and work over time. They provide us with resilience in uncertain times. My garden was a gift, the accumulation of two women's time, patience, care, and attention.

As climate chaos swirls around us, our gardens can shift to help us weather

HERBS FOR THE POLLINATORS & BUTTERFLIES

Anise Hyssop	Lilac
Aster	Mallow
Bee Balm	Marjoram
Catmint	Milkweed
Dill	Mint
False Indigo	Oregano
Goldenrod	Pansy
Lavender	Rosemary

the storms. They not only provide us with plants like chamomile to shore up our nervous systems, calendula to digest, mullein and thyme to protect our lungs from air pollution, and holy basil to grow our capacity for change but serve ecological functions as well. You can use the opportunity of growing to know the land you are standing on, save and swap seeds from your garden to share with others and to increase biodiversity, and grow extra foodstuffs to share with neighbors.

While harvesting my tulsi for winter tea, I happened upon two giant orb spiders guarding their webs. A few days earlier, I had seen three in the garden of a friend who had opened her gate to let me harvest from her bounty of yarrow. At first, I was frightened by the sight of them, as my hand had come within inches of their webs while harvesting. At once, I understood their presence as protector and gatekeeper, while they reminded me of my place and their value in our web of life. I asked if I could continue to harvest and was from then on respectful of their homes.

Growing gardens provides a haven for other life-forms. Planting a lawn grown from thyme, wild strawberries, violets, or white clovers provides nourishment for pollinators and can withstand being mowed down. In areas where wildfires are persistent, living groundcover can mitigate fires spread by embers. In the garden, the herbs we grow to be our companions can provide nourishment for other species. Plant flowers for the sake of spreading beauty and feeding pollinators. There are herbs that serve this function, too.

How do we choose what we grow? Growing a combination of medicinal plants, culinary herbs, flowers, annual vegetables, and perennial fruit is highly rewarding and can strengthen the diversity and resilience of our local ecosystems.

Growing medicinal plants from seeds might be one of my greatest joys. Whether from seed or a starter, it is a wonderful process of learning about a plant and what it takes to grow the things that nourish us. We learn how to tend, care, nourish, and support the cycles of life, death, and rebirth. The intention, the anticipation, the failure, the lessons, and the connection that unfold from growing your own medicine is by far the most rewarding.

It is important to learn what growing zone you live in, meaning the dates of your first frost and last frost, to ensure before you experiment that the plants you sow will thrive in your bioregion. You can find this information on the US Department of Agriculture (USDA) website at usda.gov. You can grow herbs in your garden among your vegetables or landscaping, you can turn your front lawn into a garden bed, you can grow herbs in pots on a kitchen windowsill or a balcony in a city apartment, or connect with a local community garden for a plot.

I also love finding medicinal plants at local farmers' markets or greenhouses and even trading with friends. A community grows around you when you begin to connect with plants in this way. If growing a plant from seed does not work for you, there are still ways to engage in the process that somehow makes that cup of lemon balm tea in the deep winter, harvested from a plant you cared for, all the more sweet. It is through the praxis of a relationship formed through tending, watering, and fending off garden pests.

These are some of my favorite medicinal plants (in alphabetical order) to grow from seed or start in a small garden or container:

- Calendula (page 138)

- California poppy

- Chamomile (page 144)

- Lavender (page 160)

- Lemon balm (page 164)

- Mint

- Rosemary (page 261)

- Sage (page 264)

- Thyme (page 272)

- Tulsi (page 198)

There are other plants that are wonderful to establish as perennials in a garden, and many can also be found through foraging. I'd like to note that while these plants are found in the Northern Hemisphere of the United States, there may be similar species growing in your bioregion, even these same ones. A tip to finding out what can grow in your region is finding out your USDA Hardiness Zone (see page 71).

- California poppy

- Elder (page 151)

- Monarda (page 175)

- Nasturtium (page 182)

- Nettle (page 117)

- Raspberry Leaf (page 254)

- Rose (page 189)

- Yarrow (page 204)

If you are looking to source your medicinal herbs, it is important to make sure they are organic and free of pesticides and other chemicals. Organic production is better not only for our bodies but for the environment, the laborers harvesting the plants, the local watersheds, the soil, and local communities as well. Locally sourced herbs are best; connect with local growers to support and help them with their "weeding." On a large scale, cultivated herbs are preferable over wild-crafted ones because you are ensuring the local population of herbs is being harvested sustainably and not solely for profit.

As we garden, we can increase biodiversity, steward native plants, and help endangered plant species find a footing again. Consider foraging for non-native invasive species like plantain, dandelion, multiflora rose, and garlic mustard and eating them, and cultivating plants like black cohosh, goldenseal, ginseng, and bloodroot in your garden. Find a list of invasive and endangered plant species in your area and see where you can help regulate the balance in your local ecosystem.

A Sacred Garden

There is a sacred art in gardening and tending to plants, which in my experience is a lifelong journey. Plants will grow. You do not need a lot of space to practice the sacred art of growing. The most important aspect to growing is a plan and preparation and a sense of curiosity and the courage to fail. You'll want to first choose a location–a balcony, a windowsill, a front yard, or a backyard. Plants can grow in so many places. Good lighting and soil are also important factors.

Observe the sun's path throughout the day: How does it stream into your home? What parts of your home and yard get the most sunlight? What is your growing zone? This will determine what types of plants will thrive in your climate. Most plants need six to eight hours of sun a day. Is your location south facing? Does it get morning shade and afternoon light? Is water easily accessible? If space is a factor, consider containers. You want a pot large enough for the plant to grow into. If you have a sunny spot, choose plants that will do well in the sun, and pick varieties for your region.

How is your soil? Is it dark and rich? You can use a home soil test kit to check for toxins, nutrients, and optimal pH. Does your soil need to be amended with compost, which is often decaying matter or animal waste? If you are growing in containers or in a raised bed, you can have more control over soil. You'll want an organic mix; I prefer organic soil mixed with mycelium, which is a key ingredient for a healthy and robust garden. If you are planting in the soil, clear and prepare the ground. Clean up weeds or consider using no-till methods of layering cardboard and three inches of soil to prepare your garden the fall before you plan to begin.

Prepare a seedling soil and mix it with water until it feels moist but not dripping wet. Place the soil into a tray or small pots or use a soil blocker. Plant two or three seeds per cell (you can thin and separate when the seedlings sprout). To water, mist the soil or water from the bottom. It often takes between five and fifteen days for seeds to germinate. Cover with a transparent dome to aid the germination process. Some plants prefer light and others prefer warm soils, so a germination mat can help facilitate the process. Set seeds in a warm spot.

CHAPTER SIX

Herbal Preparations

"The secrets are in the plants.
To elicit them you have to love them enough."

GEORGE WASHINGTON CARVER

---

*I*t is not necessary to use complex preparations and elaborate formulas to work with plants. In African American folk medicine as well as Indigenous American remedies, often only one or two herbs were used at any given time for simple preparations like teas, infusions, and decoctions. They also made vinegars, syrups, salves, juices, baths, steam inhalations, and poultices. We can incorporate plants for healing simply in our everyday lives. Among all the complicated things in our modern life, nourishment and connection can be simple. Here I explain some of the most used herbal methods that serve as a foundation in my kitchen and my apothecary. I try to infuse herbal goodness into our food in any way I can think of.

Infusions

Infusion refers simply to a water-based preparation. Think steeping herbs in water for a cup of tea or a tisane, just for longer amounts of time. An infusion is a preparation used for the flowers, leaves, and stems of a plant. Cold-water infusions are for plants like marshmallow root or hibiscus. Sun tea is an infusion from the rays and warmth of the sun.

To make an infusion, bring water to a boil; for 1 ounce of dried herbs you need 1 quart water, or for 1 tablespoon of fresh herbs use 8 ounces water. Crush the herbs in your hand or a mortar and pestle, and place them in a teapot, mug, or jar. Pour the correct amount of boiling water over your herbs, and cover the vessel to catch the volatile oils. Steep for 5 to 15 minutes for a tea. For longer, nourishing infusions, steep for up to 8 hours. Herbs like bitter chamomile need to infuse for only a few minutes. Strain the infusion in a strainer, compost the herbs, and honey to taste, if desired, and enjoy. I refrigerate my longer, nourishing infusions for up to 24 hours. Generally, nutritive plants, like violet leaf, raspberry leaf, marshmallow, or milky oats, are used for infusions.

Nettle Infusion
Nothing compares to the bright, green goodness of a nettle infusion. After a long winter, often characterized as a period of stagnation and depletion, the first spring nettles are an absolute gift from the earth.

I often use the fresh tops in cooking, as they are tender, yet as the plant grows the leaves become more tough. I dry the larger leaves to use in infusions, herbal steams, and soups. This nettle infusion is my go-to when I need a boost. Water best extracts the nutrients from the dried cell walls of a plant. To my nettle infusions, I like to add mint, apple mint, or peppermint for flavor and digestion, in addition to oat straw and fresh slices of ginger. Strain and enjoy at room temperature or cold over ice.

Decoctions

A decoction is a slower and longer simmer of bark, roots, or seeds. This method extracts constituents from tougher plant materials, like cinnamon or dandelion root. Decoctions can be ingested or used topically by soaking a cloth in the decoction for a compress. Another use for a decoction is as an herbal bath or soak. Applying an herbal tea topically is an effective and ancient way of accessing the beneficial properties of an herb.

For maximum benefit, drink 3 cups a day. For acute conditions, drink ½ cup every 30 to 60 minutes, totaling 4 cups, as needed.

To make a decoction, use 1 ounce of dried herbs per 1 quart water. Combine the herbs and water in a saucepan, cover, and bring to a boil. Lower the heat and simmer, covered, for 20 to 40 minutes. Remove from heat and strain. Drink or store in the refrigerator for 24 to 48 hours.

Honey
I adore using honey as a medium to draw out herbal constituents. The honey itself is full of wonderful properties, from being antibacterial to helping the body fight local allergens, and I try to use local, raw honey. I love to capture sweet florals in honey or to complement richer flavors like sage or thyme. Herbal honeys are often an element in drinking vinegars, added to winter teas for medicinal benefits, or used as a base for other herbal preparations, like elixirs or syrups. Electuaries are herbal honeys made with powdered herbs that are mixed right in, no straining necessary.

Vinegars
Infusing plant matter in vinegar is similar to an alcohol tincture, in which the menstruum (solvent) pulls out the plant constituents. I love using herbal infused vinegars as the base for salad dressings,

for drinking vinegars, for cleaning, and for hair rinses.

Raw apple cider vinegar (ACV) helps promote digestion by encouraging growth of good bacteria. ACV supports the immune system, inflammation, and digestion. Topically, it can be used for cuts, abrasions, skin funguses, and rashes. Herbal vinegars are best made with dried herbs for the most potent extraction. The juice from fresh herbs can water down the vinegar before it can extract the plants' constituents. You can use crushed dried herbs or powdered herbs for more potent herbal vinegars. If you are looking for a simpler culinary vinegar, fresh herbs can be used.

To make a vinegar, chop the dried herb or grind it in a mortar and pestle. Fill a clean jar a quarter of the way with the herb. Pour apple cider vinegar over the herb until the jar is full. Either use a plastic lid or place a square of parchment paper over the jar and secure it with a metal lid. Store in a cool, dark place, shaking it daily, for 14 days or half a moon cycle: full moon to new moon or new moon to full moon. Strain the vinegar through cheesecloth into another clean, sterilized jar. Label and store it in a cool dark place or refrigerate for up to 6 months.

Take 1 teaspoon of vinegar up to three times a day when needed, added to water, tea, or oil (to make a vinaigrette).

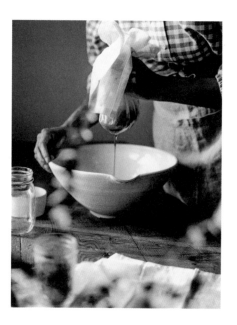

Herbal Infused Oils

Infused oils are perfect for self-massage, a nourishing act of self-care. Herbal oils can help relieve tension and inflammation and lubricate the joints. Our skin is also our largest organ, and we can absorb herbal oil through our skin. What we put on our bodies matter. If you've ever carried self-hatred or self-doubt, self-massage can help you appreciate yourself in an intentional way. It is also a lovely way to connect with a partner, loved one, or child. My favorite oil for little ones is chamomile or lavender; rub it on the bottoms of their feet to calm them before bedtime.

There are two ways to make herb-infused oils.

Folk Method

Use 1 ounce of dried herbs to 12 fluid ounces of the carrier oil of your choice (see Choice of Carrier Oils, opposite).

Grind the herbs well in a mortar and pestle or crumble them with your hands. Fill a dry sterilized jar halfway with the herbs. Pour the carrier oil over the herbs to the top, making sure all the herbs are covered. Use a clean spoon to stir the mixture thoroughly. Cover with a square of wax paper and a metal lid, or use a plastic lid. Shake the oil in between your hands infusing it with your healing intention.

Place the jar in a dark, warm spot for 4 to 6 weeks—or a full lunar cycle from new moon to new moon. Every few days, shake the jar. Decant the oil by straining it through an organic muslin or cheesecloth and strainer, squeezing the remainder of the oils out. Pour the oil into a clean, sterilized jar to let it settle. Strain again a few days later and pour the infused oil into an amber jar and label it. Store in a cool, dark place. Herbal oils can remain potent for 6 months to a year.

Stovetop Method

Place a small amount of water in the bottom of a double boiler; you do not want water boiling up and touching the oil. (Alternatively, use a large pot that easily holds a smaller bowl or pot.) Using 1 ounce dried herbs to 12 fluid ounces of your choice of carrier oil, combine them in the smaller pot. Set the pots over very low heat for 4 to 8 hours. Remove the pots from the heat, let the infused oil cool, decant into a dry sterilized jar as described in the folk method above, and label. The oil can also be infused in a slow cooker or a heat-safe jar in a few inches of water, placing a few lids under the jar to protect it from direct heat.

Salves

Salves are a balm made from an herbal-infused carrier oil and beeswax. I often use cocoa butter or shea butter to create a softer consistency. Salves can be used for dry winter skin, bruises, burns, muscle aches, relaxation, and wounds. They are one of my go-to remedies (see page 289).

Syrups

Essentially, a syrup is an herbal infusion or decoction that is reduced and added to honey or another sweetener to extend its shelf life, for example, mix a syrup from one or two parts decoction to two parts sweetener. You can also add alcohol to make it more shelf stable. The most popular syrup is elderberry (see page 232).

Poultice

This traditional preparation of herbs crushed in water is made into a paste, then spread on a cloth and applied directly to the body. It is commonly used with hot water and a hot cloth to ease pain and relax tissues. A cold poultice can be applied to burns and inflamed skin conditions. Commonly used poultice herbs include plantain for bee stings and bug bites, violet leaf for sunburns, or yarrow and calendula as a vulnerary for rashes and skin eruptions.

CHOICE OF CARRIER OILS

Almond oil: This light oil isn't too greasy on the skin. It's great for all skin types and works well as a massage oil.

- -

Coconut oil: Although it can feel greasy to the touch, it's very moisturizing to dry skin and hair and has antibacterial properties.

- -

Grapeseed oil: This oil is more highly refined, but it's toning and nongreasy. It also extracts components from plants effectively.

- -

Jojoba oil: A good oil for acne-prone skin, this is balancing and soothing for inflamed skin, such as sunburns.

- -

Olive oil: Commonly used olive oil can be greasy, but it's soothing for dry, damaged, and inflamed skin and hair.

- -

Shea butter: Use this for a creamier texture and to protect the skin.

- -

Sunflower oil: A common oil that is often available locally, it has a light texture, is nongreasy, and can be used on many skin types.

HERBAL CONSTITUENTS

Alkaloids
ACTIONS: antispasmodic, bitter, emmenagogue, galactagogue, nervine, sedative, stimulant.

EXAMPLES: borage, coffee, goldenseal. Most soluble in alcohol, glycerin, vinegar.

Bitters
ACTIONS: antimicrobial, cholagogue, cooling, digestive stimulant, hepatic (liver) laxative, nervine.

EXAMPLES: angelica root, dandelion leaf and root, chamomile flower, yarrow (aerial parts). Most soluble in water, alcohol, vinegar, glycerin.

Flavonoids
(pigments in brightly colored plants; occur as glycosides or without a sugar molecule)

ACTIONS: anticancer, anti-inflammatory, antioxidant, antispasmodic, antiviral, cardiotonic, diuretic, hypotensive.

EXAMPLES: hawthorn leaf, fruit, and flower; turmeric; tea; chamomile flower; red clover (aerial parts). Most soluble in water.

Glycosides
(constituents with a sugar combined with a non-sugar compound; some glycosides can be toxic and must be used carefully)

ACTIONS: antifungal, anti-inflammatory, antimicrobial, bitter, cardiotonic, cardioactive, laxative.

EXAMPLES: yellow dock, hawthorn leaf, flower and fruit. Most soluble in water, alcohol, vinegar, glycerin.

Mucilages
ACTIONS: anti-inflammatory, demulcent, emollient, laxative.

EXAMPLES: aloe leaf, marshmallow root and leaf, plantain leaf and seed. Most soluble in cool water.

Polysaccharides
(complex carbohydrates)

ACTIONS: immunomodulating, nutritive.

EXAMPLES: astragalus root, burdock root, echinacea root, reishi mushroom, shiitake mushroom. Most soluble in hot water.

- -

Resins
(sticky substances that form from the oxidation of volatile oils)

ACTIONS: antimicrobial, antispasmodic, bitter, expectorant, relaxing, stimulating, vulnerary.

EXAMPLES: calendula flower, hops, pine. Most soluble in alcohol, warm oil.

- -

Saponins
(types of glycosides that contain a fat-soluble base joined to a water-soluble sugar; molecules create detergent; some saponins are toxic)

ACTIONS: adaptogenic, anticancer, anti-inflammatory, antispasmodic, diuretic, expectorant, hepatoprotective, hormone modulating, immunomodulating.

EXAMPLES: chickweed (aerial parts), licorice root. Most soluble in water, glycerin, alcohol.

- -

Tannins
(polyphenolic compounds that contract and dry tissues by binding with and precipitating proteins)

ACTIONS: anti-diarrheal, anti-inflammatory, antimicrobial, astringent, diuretic, hemostatic.

EXAMPLES: plantain leaf, raspberry leaf, rose petal, willow bark and leaf, witch hazel leaf and bark, yarrow aerial parts. Most soluble in glycerin, water, vinegar, alcohol.

- -

Volatile Oils
(unstable aromatic compounds that volatilize easily)

ACTIONS: antimicrobial, circulatory, decongestant, diffusive, nervine, stimulant.

EXAMPLES: aniseed, ginger, lavender bud, lemon balm, peppermint leaf, rosemary, sage, tea tree leaf, valerian root. Most soluble in alcohol, oil, fat.

Herbal Actions and Energetics

Herbal actions are the specific effects a plant has on a body. Herbs can have multiple actions. Herbal properties are the qualities of a plant and the constituents found in the plant.

- **ADAPTOGENS** support the body from external stress, enhancing immunity and the body's ability to adapt to changing landscapes. They enable the body to maintain balance through stressful shifts in the environment.

- **ALTERATIVES** work generally to tonify the body's systems involved in nutrient assimilation and detoxification. They promote the elimination of waste through the kidneys, liver, colon, skin, and lungs.

- **ANALGESICS** reduce the sensation of pain perceived by the brain.

- **ANTIFUNGALS** help kill or limit funguses.

- **ANTI-INFLAMMATORIES** help reduce inflammation or keep it at bay.

- **ANTISEPTICS** help the body kill microbes on its external surfaces.

- **ANTISPASMODICS** prevent or ease spasms and cramps in the muscles, reducing physical tension and easing psychological tension. They can also relax and smooth tissues. Antispasmodics calm the autonomic nervous system, not the central nervous system, so they don't have a sedative effect.

- **ANTIVIRALS** help the body fight viruses (e.g., lemon balm, sumac).

- **APHRODISIACS** increase libido, potency, and sexual pleasure (e.g., hibiscus, rose).

- **AROMATICS** are used as nervines and expectorants. They are high in volatile oils with a fragrant aroma (e.g., lavender).

- **ASTRINGENTS** tighten the tissues. Think about how your mouth puckers when you drink a cup of tea; this is astringency in action. It is caused by tannins, a group of complex chemicals. When applied externally, an astringent stanches bleeding, and internally it can stop hemorrhaging. These are important in healing wounds and in the digestive system (e.g., elderflower, rose).

- **BITTERS** taste bitter and ease or stimulate digestion (e.g., chamomile, dandelion).

- **CARMINATIVES** ease spasms in the digestive system (e.g., cinnamon, lemon balm).

- **DIAPHORETICS** promote perspiration (e.g., elderflower, yarrow).

- **DIURETICS** increase the flow of urine from the body (e.g., dandelion).

- **EMMENAGOGUES** stimulate and normalize the menstrual flow or tonify the female reproductive system (e.g., calendula, ginger, juniper, raspberry leaf, rosemary, yarrow).

- **EMOLLIENTS** are applied to skin to smooth and soften or protect it (e.g., chickweed, mallow, mullein, plantain).

- **EXPECTORANTS** help and support the body in clearing the lungs and respiratory tract.

- **HEPATICS** affect the liver and functions of the liver.

- **NERVINES** tone the nervous system, either stimulating, sedating, or relaxing it (e.g., chamomile, lavender, lemon balm, peppermint, red clover, rosemary).

- **NUTRITIVES** are foods, like herbs, that are very safe for daily consumption and provide nourishing and tonic minerals.

- **STIMULANTS** quicken and enliven the physiological functions of the body (cardamom, cinnamon, garlic, juniper, peppermint, rosemary, sage, yarrow).

- **TONICS** strengthen the body through specific affinities to organ systems or the whole body (burdock, calendula, chamomile, dandelion, elecampane, garlic, hawthorn, nettles, oats, raspberry leaf).

- **VULNERARIES** aid and promote wound healing when applied externally, used internally as well (aloe, burdock, calendula, elder, garlic, mullein, plantain, St. John's wort, thyme, witch hazel, yarrow).

KITCHEN APOTHECARY TOOLKIT

Here is a list of items needed for simple foraging and making herbal preparations in your kitchen.

Amber dropper bottles	Hori hori or foraging knife	Mortar and pestle
Foraging or identification guide	Kitchen scale	Organic muslin or cheesecloth
Funnel	Kitchen shears	Spice grinder
Gathering baskets	Mason jars	Strainer

Pantry Items

Alcohol	Beeswax	Salt
Almond oil	Grapeseed oil	Shea butter
Aloe vera gel	Olive oil	
Apple cider vinegar	Raw or local honey	

Herbal Energetics

Energetics describe the subtle yet profound ways a plant impacts the body, mind, or spirit. Understanding herbal tastes is one of our most important skills when working within the plant realm. Taste is a vital aspect in traditional Chinese medicine (TCM), Western herbalism, and Ayurveda. Our ancestors relied on taste to give them information about what was safe to eat and what was not. We use our senses to interact with the world, and it is through herbal energetics that we gain information on how a plant works in our body. It is considered in terms of temperature, moisture, and tension and can also refer to the tissue states in the body.

Tastes stimulate our nervous system, especially the enteric nervous system of the stomach or the gastric nerves, increasing digestive fire. In Ayurveda, there are generally six tastes: *sweet, sour, salt, pungent, bitter, and astringent*. There are also herbal energetics that help us understand how herbs affect our body: cooling, drying, stimulating, warming, relaxing, and moistening. We can use Ayurveda and TCM to understand balance, yin and yang, and apply them to Western herbs.

Know and trust your sources of herbs and obtain organic when possible. Take care when using herbs long term and in potent formulas. Use caution and discernment when using herbs in pregnancy, with young children, and with liver or kidney disease; when using prescription medications, use the supervision of a qualified and experienced professional. Do not take essential oils internally.

Toxic Herbs

Some herbs can be highly toxic and should be taken with extreme caution in very small doses and only under the guidance of a trained professional, if at all.

Not all herbs are plants to work with for healing and medicine. They may be plants to work with in a spiritual or ritualized nature. You may notice some of your favorite flower species are toxic, which means they are not meant to be used internally and/or topically. Arnica (*Arnica montana*), for instance, is a plant in the Asteraceae family often used in formulas for muscle aches and pains, but it is not to be consumed internally. Foxglove (*Digitalis* spp.) is a flower I adore growing from seed in my garden, but it is toxic to ingest. With plants, it is important to exercise caution as you are learning. Our ancestors who worked with plants had intimate knowledge about which ones were safe and which were not, and they used those distinctions to their advantage. Pokeweed, for instance, is a toxic plant, but there are recorded cases of its usage in African American herbalism.

- Arnica (*Arnica montana*)*

- Belladonna, deadly nightshade (*Atropa belladonna*)

- Dogbane (*Rauwolfia* spp.)

- Foxglove (*Digitalis* spp.)

- Greater celandine (*Chelidonium majus*)

- Henbane (*Hyoscyamus niger*)

- Jimsonweed, devil's snare (*Datura stramonium*)

- Lily of the valley (*Convallaria majuscula*)

- Mandrake (*Mandragora officinarum*)

- Mayapple (*Podophyllum peltatum*)

- Monkshood (*Aconitum* spp.)

- Opium poppy (*Papaver somniferum*)

- Poke (*Phytolacca americana*)

- Poison ivy (*Toxicodendron radicans*)

- Pulsatilla, pasque flower (*Pulsatilla vulgaris*)

- Quinine (*Cinchona* spp.)

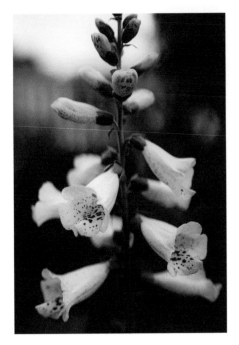

*Arnica can be safely used topically.

Plants work differently with different people and even in different seasons of our lives. That is why it becomes important to understand energetics and to truly listen to your body's needs, which I believe we are not adequately taught or encouraged to do. Pregnancy is one season in which you want to go slow with plants and use tried-and-true safe herbs and consult your health-care practitioner.

The first three groups of herbs on this list can damage a developing fetus, while all of them have the potential to cause miscarriage. Stimulants can also lower birth weight. To be sure, the following herbs should never be used in pregnancy.

- Aloe (*Aloe vera*)

- Barberry (*Berberis* spp.)

- Black cohosh (*Actaea racemosa*)

- Blue cohosh (*Caulophyllum thalictroides*)

- Goldenseal (*Hydrastis canadensis*)

- Greater celandine (*Chelidonium majus*)

- Juniper (*Juniperus communis*)

- Mugwort (*Artemisia vulgaris*)

- Motherwort (*Leonurus cardiaca*)

- Oregano (*Origanum vulgare*)

- Oregon grape (*Berberis aquifolium*)

- Pennyroyal (*Mentha pulegium*)

- Pokeweed (*Phytolacca americana*)

- Quinine (*Cinchona* spp.)

- Rosemary (*Rosmarinus officinalis*)

- Rue (*Ruta graveolens*)

- Sage (*Salvia officinalis*)

- Tansy (*Tanacetum vulgare*)

- Thuja (*Thuja occidentalis*)

- Wormwood (*Artemisia absinthium*)

Safe herbs for pregnancy include chamomile, echinacea, ginger, nettle, oat, and raspberry leaf.

As we dive into the experiential practice of working with plants within the seasonal rhythms, we can begin to apply and understand some of the concepts covered in the previous chapters. I hope my personal story and the introduction of intuitive herbalism has piqued your curiosity about how plants can come into your own daily practices. Within each season, there are monographs for plants you might grow or forage, and there are food recipes, herbal beverages, and herbal remedies to help you incorporate the plants more broadly. I once had my good friend and herbal mentor Rachel tell me to choose one plant to befriend each season. I encourage you to do the same: pick one plant, learn its name, its energetics, and its song, and see if you get along. Try to incorporate it in many ways over many days to see if its energetics align with yours. This is not a process to rush but an invitation into a lifelong journey of living with and for the earth.

PART THREE

Seasonal Wisdom, Herbal Recipes & Plant Monographs

*P*lants offer our bodies support not only through their biochemical properties, but their energetics and psychological and spiritual nature as well. I have accessed so much healing through aligning with the seasonal rhythms of the earth. When I work with the flow of my own inner cycles, the phases of the moon, and take cues from the cyclical nature of the earth and the seasons around me, it all becomes a portal to deeper awareness of myself, the earth, and our inherent bond. I exist in a flow. We can move through collective and personal trauma through practicing ritual and deep relationship with the plant world.

We are deeply influenced by our environments, and our environment, in turn, is directly and indirectly impacted by our actions. It is imperative we proceed with more intention and relatedness to help combat the climate crisis. When we are aware of what is moving through our bodies, we can in turn act with more awareness and intention in our day-to-day lives.

Aligning with the moon phases and the seasons shifts, honoring the seasons of our lives, opens our perception and deepens our understanding of our humanity. In this section, I highlight simple rituals, herbal recipes, and seasonal rhythms and practices to attune to the plants that arrive in each season. I share how our bodies' energetics shift by the season, where to focus our psyche, and plant allies to befriend in times of need. I share ways to preserve and prepare plants in multiple manners, to enjoy immediately or to put up for the seasons ahead. I want to illuminate the alchemy possible in the present moment. This is an invitation to discover the abundance and creativity existing in the now and transform it into healing and connection through food, foraging, cultivating plants, seasonal rhythms, and rituals. With each turn of the wheel of time, the change in season, cycle of the moon, and movement of the stars, we are given an opening to move closer to wholeness, not the myth of perfection. Embracing our light and dark, our joy and our fears, our inherited wounds, and our inherent light.

Seasonal living is enlivening, because each cycle is a period of refinement, an opportunity to try again, to shift, to change, transform, and heal. Each season is a chance to embody learned wisdom from past failures and successes, allowing that to inform the present moment. Our built world reflects the natural world: the word *month* takes its roots from "moon." A month originally had 29 to 30 days to mirror the lunar cycle.

> *"Greed subsumes love and compassion; living simply makes room for them. Living simply is the primary way everyone can resist greed every day. . . . It is the way we learn to practice compassion, daily affirming our connection to a world community."*

BELL HOOKS

Living Simply, Living Slow

Slow living is not an excuse to stop paying attention or spiritually bypass the harm perpetuated by humans. In fact, in my mind, it is quite the opposite: it gives us the opportunity to pause and look more closely. It is in the action of slowing down that we can see the ripple effects and consequences, both positive and negative, of our thoughts, our beliefs, our actions, and the impact they have on us, our families, our communities, other vulnerable communities and people, and the health of our planet. Slowing down should not be an excuse to live in a homogeneous bubble but the opportunity to investigate and become curious.

Slow living is an invitation to disentangle our lives, as best as we can as individuals, from trying to assert our ego over others and to understand the oneness of our existence. The intimacy to know with more clarity when you are hurting, marginalized, and oppressed, so am I. When the earth, the land, the waterways, the soil is depleted and polluted, so am I. To em-

body equity means when I rise, I am holding your hand, and when you fall, I fall, too. When we slow down, we understand that turning a blind eye is an act of negligence. Slow living is not black and white; it is a continual process and movement of examining and reexamining. I think we should all be asking ourselves "why" more often.

Slow living inspires intentionality. Rooting into the seasons inspires presence and experience to counter the narrative born from capitalism's exponential growth models. In nature, there is no linear timeline and forward progress. Life is cyclical. In nature all things are conceived, born, grow, languish, and die to replenish the soil of collective existence. Rest is a radical act.

We will not be perfect in our journeys. Perfectionism is a device of the oppressor, a paradigm that limits our creativity and ability to dream up new ways of existing on this earth. Individual action alone will never accomplish our goals. We are a whole, and when we act as such, we will see much more change.

Folk cultures respected and had reverence for the earth, honoring the cycles of nature, living, death and rebirth, our creation stories. Old religions had goddesses of creation—the ultimate representation of the feminine. Putting back this sacred connection, respect for and understanding of what gives us life.

Let us reclaim our roots, our worth, deep regard, and reverence for ourselves and others. Let us reclaim the sacred space and safety to embody what it means to be human. To allow spoken word to sink into our skin, to allow the beauty of the natural world to flow through us to create art, to embody wholly the pleasure and pain of this experience on earth, which we know is finite, ever changing and shifting.

When we take a deep, slow breath, we activate the relaxation response. We can find presence in this moment and open to space of possibility.

Dance and Sing Your Joy

When we are rested, when we have acknowledged ourselves, we can be more ready to share in our own joy and the joy of others.

Invite kindred spirits and disparate souls to our table, to our gardens, providing them a seat to understand each other more deeply and connect to the humanity within us all. When we make space within ourselves, we have more capacity to hold space for others. Love is action. The masks we willingly and unknowingly wear keep us from connecting and showing true vulnerability. Plants help us take off our masks to sit with more ease in the uncomfortable nature of vulnerability. When we share our pain, our expression with others, they can let us know we are not alone. When we can break through the shells of our conditioning, we can find ripe soil ready to grow new ways of being.

Cups, bowls, glasses, clinking of jars on the pantry shelves. These are our well-worn instruments and vessels that hold centuries of healing, our tools to work our magic. We alchemize the elements: fire, water, earth, and air. They are our ingredients to heal and create and honor the seasons of our lives. The daily work of healing requires our devotion, the dressing and undressing, the tending to our wounds. Prepare the cup of tea, make it an elaborate ritual, pour yourself into the moment. See the steam rising, bless the herbs, thank the bees for the sweetness of their honey, and stir it all together, imbuing it with your deepest intentions and gratitude. In this alchemy, you will find magic in the mundane and bless your life with your every action.

We've forgotten our craft; we've lost our way. We cannot leave the magic and the healing work to others to do for us. Some of us were never taught, others have had our ways beaten out of us, others assimilated out of safety. But still in the safety of our kitchen, we continued to use our hearts and hands to heal. It reverberates in our bones. Let us follow the sweet hum of the forest, the dance of the prairies, to the root, rock, leaf and flower back to our bones.

We can dance off the heaviness, summon the power of our voice through song, and find joy in the healing that unfolds over time. In modern times of overwhelm, we can call in the ancient and time-tested ways to move the body, spirit and mind. The seasons can offer a sense of normalcy when things feel awry. Let us humble ourselves to receive the stories of plants. The plants and the natural world help us remember our medicine. I want to invite you to get quiet enough, to become moved by the spirit of curiosity to learn their songs for yourself.

The plants hold sweetness, nourishment, and guidance on dark days. Too much of anything can be poison, too little, ineffective; just right is the medicine. Use plants every day if you can. You don't need to only turn to plants in desperation but find the right relationship with plants through humility, devotion, and practice.

The basis of my work is to encourage others to deepen their ties to earth and season to locate a sense of belonging beyond social constructs. Wherever you stand and whoever you are, you deserve a meaningful relationship with our Earth. This reciprocal relationship imparts a sense of well-being through soothing our nervous system, allowing us the space to feel safe.

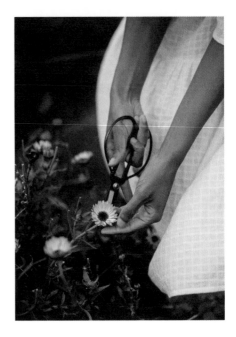

We can cultivate belonging, reciprocity, resilience and regard through cultivating plants, foraging for plants, crafting with our hands and hearts and sharing meals. After I recovered from an eating disorder, food was still a love language, and engaging with food in a balanced, nourishing, and fun way is healing. I try to not restrict myself to make foods off limits, and to cook with whole, organic, and local foods as much as possible. Food nourishes our body and soul. Food is a way we create and nurture our stories. Food brings people and plants together in an alchemy of sorts.

When we sit with plants, when we listen, when we offer our regard to their intelligence and life forms, we open ourselves to be filled with their lessons, their healing, their wisdom collected for millennia.

Spring

Emergence
Spring, stem and leaves

Astrology of spring
Aries (cardinal fire), Taurus (fixed earth),
Gemini (mutable air)

Energetics
Wet becoming hot

Direction
East, when the sun rises, infancy,
the birth of the sun each day, the morning,
new beginnings, a waxing moon

Chakra
Sacral

*A Season of
Blossom, Bark,
and Leaves*

*Waxing
Crescent Moon*

*Fertility, Birth,
Renewal*

*East, Where the
Sun Is Reborn
Each Morning*

"In the spring, at the end of the day, you should smell like dirt."

MARGARET ATWOOD

S pring is a reminder that life is filled with second, third, fourth chances. Seasons are to begin again, to try again, to turn a page. We can begin again with each turn of the wheel of time.

Late winter to early spring is a time characterized in traditional Chinese medicine as carrying the energy of damp stagnation. Energy is rising from the root. We prepare the soil and nourish the root chakra. Here in the Northern Hemisphere, the robin returns because, as the ground thaws after a long winter's sleep, frozen ground turns to mud and the earth slowly warms and awakens. Earthworms wriggle and sap begins to flow in the warm days and cool nights under the full Worm Moon (Indigenous Americans call the March full moon rising Worm Moon or Sap Moon). The warming daytime sun and cold nights mean sap is beginning to flow.

Beside thawing creeks, pussy willow blooms and blue skies peek through. On our woodland walks, snowdrops emerge, and bits of green are spotted—garlic mustard, young nettle tops. The liminal space between winter and spring is a hard time for me. I experience impatience and anticipation to begin again. Yet the season of spring asks for our patience, much like a mother waiting to give birth. The

plants arrive on their own schedule, there may be a second or third "last snow," and the lessons available in spring are ones of observations, planning, cultivating, and preparation. It is a season unto itself to honor what is coming, what is going, and to prepare the heart and mind. In spring our energy, thoughts, and actions turn outward as we venture out of hibernation.

As our ancestors looked to the sky for cues about time, as the earth rotated, the appearance of the Pleiades in the sky, also known as the Seven Sisters, signaled the beginning of the planting season. The full Flower Moon shines bright in the evening sky and the earth is in full bloom.

The spring equinox, arriving around March 21, welcomes balance, equal night and day. The earth and all its inhabitants bask in the increasing light and warmth as the sun returns. But the questions still stand: What darkness do we need to confront to make our hearts ready for new life? What decay in relationships, emotions, and patterns need to be composted to make room for growth and expansion?

How can we carry the lessons distilled over winter, the dark night of our soul? How can we channel and use our imaginations to envision what comes next? Out of the soil, darkness, and muck comes renewal. What stirs within you?

The crocus and the jonquil declare April is here, and in a fury, I begin to spring clean: the garden bed, our home, my body. After months of being shut, I open windows for a gust of fresh air, to say farewell to the detritus and stagnation built up after a long winter. I pull on my muck boots for long, slow walks around the garden, staring at the muddy piles of melting snow for signs of the perennials who join the garden year after year. Wait until days are above fifty degrees to clear beds of the debris of gardens past, as beneficial insects are still wintering in the leaves and hollowed-out stems. But could it be time to tuck cold-hardy seedlings in the soil? April's Pink Moon, the Budding Moon, brings renewal, a burst of life and rebirth. The spring greens offer their medicine after a long winter to move stagnation, to wake up our bodies, and to cleanse, clear, and detoxify. The light has shifted ever so slightly, and our hens begin to lay eggs again with the extra moments of sun.

Spring cleaning can take many forms. We tuck away woolen winter clothes and donate what no longer suits our purposes. Make rituals from sweeping and washing the floors, dusting the cobwebs from the corners of your mind and home, opening windows to let the air element bring in fresh life, placing fresh-cut flowers in your room, ritual baths.

In May, life blooms. Fiddlehead ferns unfurl and woodland ephemerals emerge; bloodroot, trillium, and rue signal mushrooms are fruiting bodies are near. Sunlight and rainy days nurture the leaves to grow. The gravity of the waxing moon pulls shoots and leaves from the ground and beckons blossoms on the trees. Harvest rhubarb when crabapple blossoms. Asparagus, radishes, and nettles abound; magnolia buds burst and strawberry blossoms. Fertile, creative energy flows.

GATHER: Sap for maple syrup, fresh nettle tops, and garlic mustard in March; violets and dandelion flowers, pussy willow and forsythia branches to decorate the table in April; asparagus, rhubarb, and nettles to dry in May.

MAKE: Pesto, warming dandelion chai, nourishing infusions to restore depleted energy and revive the spirit in March; wild greens frittatas. Rhubarb shrubs, lilac syrup, floral jellies in May.

DO: Tuck spring seeds into the soil, collect the snowdrops and violets and press them between pages of a book. Move your body with intention. Emerge from hibernation and connect with neighbors. Take woodland walks and mushroom hunt, identify spring ephemeral flowers, indulge in floral baths.

Dandelion TARAXACUM OFFICINALE

A perennial plant, dandelions grow through the cracks of sidewalks and persist despite being trampled and scorned. With a resilient energy, they are found in lawns and roadsides, in the cracks of city sidewalks and in disturbed soils. Dandelion helps one connect with the courage to grow tall despite it all. Eat dandelions before trying to eradicate them with chemicals and pesticides.

After long winters, I imagine dandelions, known for their deep and bitter nutritious greens, were once greeted with smiling faces and eager hearts. As a nutritive and alterative herb, it contains vitamins A, B, C, and E, potassium, iron, magnesium, calcium, and zinc. Dandelion greens in spring help my seasonal anemia. Wild foods are abundant and contain more minerals than food produced in the nutrient-depleted soils of our contemporary agricultural systems. Mixing in small amounts of dandelion greens with other greens adds nutrition and balances out the bitter flavor.

Dandelion flowers can be baked into cookies and cakes or made into wine and tea as a digestive tonic. The leaves are bitter, so soaking the leaves in salt water before sautéing can help; then cook them like other greens. Dandelion is a diuretic and aids kidney function and is best consumed young. The root is bitter when harvested in the spring and in the fall has more inulin, a polysaccharide and dietary fiber that benefits gut health. Roots can be dug, sliced, dried

in the oven or dehydrator, and made into beverages. Dandelion is a welcome friend in our garden, and I encourage you to make friends, too.

When one is grasping onto old anger and cannot release rage, dandelion flower essence helps clear and move you through the anger. Dandelion root biochemically stimulates bile flow, clears heat, and cleanses the liver, supporting emotional release. In traditional Chinese medicine, the liver is said to hold the emotions of anger. Anger is often a secondary emotion protecting our vulnerable selves. The sunshine yellow of dandelion imparts the hope of the sun. In releasing stress and stagnant emotions, one can finally experience a sense of effortlessness and rest. Ease comes when one can release the rigidity held in the body and the mind.

The spirit of dandelion flower essence can support one who feels the need to control and demand from others because they feel out of control. This balance allows one to exist with more harmony and ease.

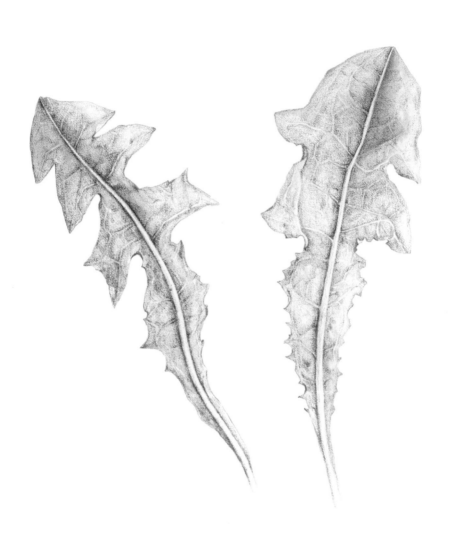

Plant family
Asteraceae

Other names
Lion's tooth, pisanli in Haitian Kreyòl (meaning "urinate the bed" because of it diuretic actions)

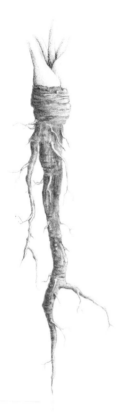

Region
Dandelions are native to Eurasia. Growing in temperate regions, they have been introduced and spread to North and South America, India, Australia, and Europe, following the footsteps of human migration.

Botanical description
Yellow ray florets and petals. Each flower head is a composite of many smaller flowers. The dandelion has a thick taproot that reaches deep into the soil. Hollow stalk with milky liquid, irregular toothed and serrated leaves.

Herbal actions
Astringent, bitter, diuretic, nutritive, digestive stimulant, alterative, hepatic, tonic

---

Energetics
Cooling, bitter, and drying

Flower essence
Compels you to be here now

Gather
The young leaves and dig bitter roots in the spring; flowers in spring and summer (though the leaves may be more bitter); roots in the fall will be sweeter. Make sure to harvest from plants free of pesticides and contaminated soils.

Grow
USDA Hardiness Zone 3 to 10. Enjoys morning sun but will grow anywhere. Can be started indoors 6 weeks before the last frost, prefers cool soils. Plant seeds ⅛ inch deep; germinates in 7 to 14 days.

Preparations
Bitters, vinegars, decoctions, wine, baked goods, infused oils, eaten raw, roots stir-fried.

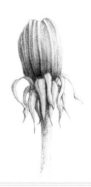

Spring Cleansing Tonic

This spring tonic nourishes and cleanses the blood after a long winter. I find when I'm feeling depleted, I add 2 tablespoons to plant-based milk and ice cubes for a refreshing and nourishing beverage. It maintains my energy levels when I go about my day. I love the addition of molasses to this recipe, an iron-rich ingredient used widely in African American herbal remedies. I look for these dried ingredients in the bulk herbs at my local co-op or order them from a reputable herbal store.

1 tablespoon
dried yellow dock root

1 tablespoon
dried dandelion root

1 tablespoon
dried burdock root

1 tablespoon
dried astragalus root

2 tablespoons dried rose hips

1 teaspoon cardamom pods

3 tablespoons
dried nettle leaf

1 cup molasses

*Makes
1 quart
jar*

Combine the yellow dock, dandelion, burdock, astragalus, rose hips, cardamom, and 8 cups water in a pot. Set on low heat and simmer the herbs, uncovered, for 30 to 45 minutes, stirring occasionally, until almost reduced by half. Do not boil but keep the herbs at a low simmer. This is your decoction. Remove the pot from the heat, stir in the nettle leaf, and let sit for 10 to 15 minutes, strain, and then stir in the molasses. Let the syrup cool and pour it into bottles.

Dosage: Take 1 tablespoon one to three times per day. I often like to add this to a cup of warm nondairy milk for a little midmorning beverage.

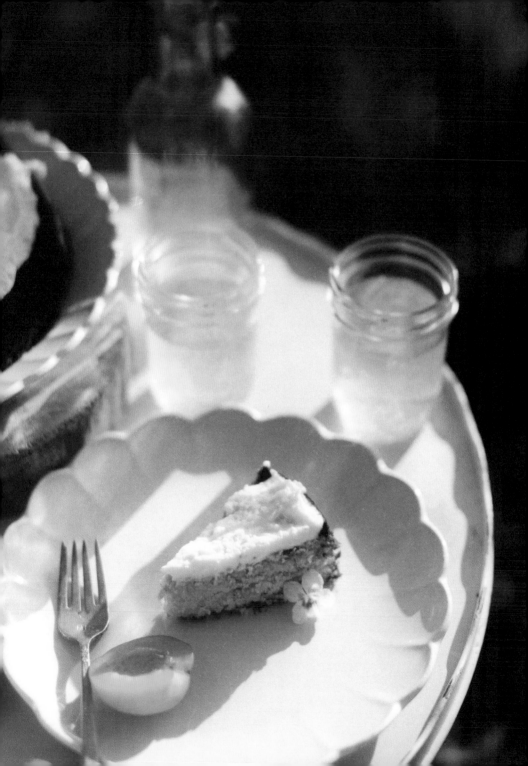

Dandelion Almond Cake with Lilac Mascarpone Frosting

This recipe is a marriage between two of my favorite recipes: lemon–olive oil cake and cornbread. I use almond and cornmeal here for an earthy texture. This cake is moist and dense with a hint of floral sweetness from the lilac syrup in the frosting. The lilac syrup can be swapped for other floral syrups, sugar, or maple. The sprinkle of dandelion petals makes this the ideal spring cake and drops me into the present moment.

Makes 10 to 12 servings

Preheat the oven to 350°F. In a bowl, sift together the almond flour, cornmeal, tapioca flour, baking powder, and salt. In a separate bowl, beat the butter, olive oil, honey, and vanilla. Whisk in the eggs, one at a time, until blended. Stir in the Greek yogurt, lemon zest, and dandelion petals. Fold in the flours. Pour batter into a greased and floured 9-inch springform pan, smooth the top, and bake for 45 minutes, until a skewer inserted in the center comes out clean and the cake is golden.

Remove from the oven and let cool before icing.

1½ cups almond flour

1½ cups cornmeal

¼ cup tapioca flour

1 teaspoon baking powder

½ teaspoon salt

¾ cup (1½ sticks) unsalted butter

3 tablespoons olive oil

1 cup honey

2 teaspoons vanilla extract

3 large eggs

½ cup Greek yogurt

Zest of 1 lemon

2 cups dandelion petals separated from the greens

Lilac Mascarpone Frosting

Lilac Mascarpone Frosting

Combine all the ingredients in a stand mixer, bowl, or jar. Using a whisk attachment on a stand mixer or on an immersion blender, whip the ingredients until soft peaks form. Refrigerate until ready to use.

¾ cup heavy cream

½ cup mascarpone cheese

3 tablespoons Lilac Syrup (page 114)

Pinch of salt

Sweetener to taste (optional)

Dandelion Coffee

*Roasted dandelion root can make a warming spring beverage
paired with carminative spices. I make a batch of this for
when I'm in the garden planting spring crops and listening
to the birdsong. This coffee alternative, with its roasted and
earthy flavors, helps you stay grounded. When you find you
are overtaken by anger about the state of the world and need
to drop into your body and into the moment, dandelion is
your ally.*

*Makes 2
servings*

Combine the filtered water, ginger, dandelion root, peppercorns, clove, cinnamon, and vanilla in a saucepan. Cover the pan, bring it just to a boil, then turn down the heat and simmer for 10 minutes. Strain the mixture into a mug. Add milk to the same saucepan to heat it, whisking or frothing it, stir in the honey, pour into dandelion coffee, and drink immediately.

12 ounces filtered water

½-inch ginger slice

1 teaspoon ground, roasted
dandelion root

2 black peppercorns

1 whole clove

¼ teaspoon ground cinnamon

¼ teaspoon vanilla extract

1 cinnamon stick

½ cup milk (your choice)

1 tablespoon honey
or maple syrup

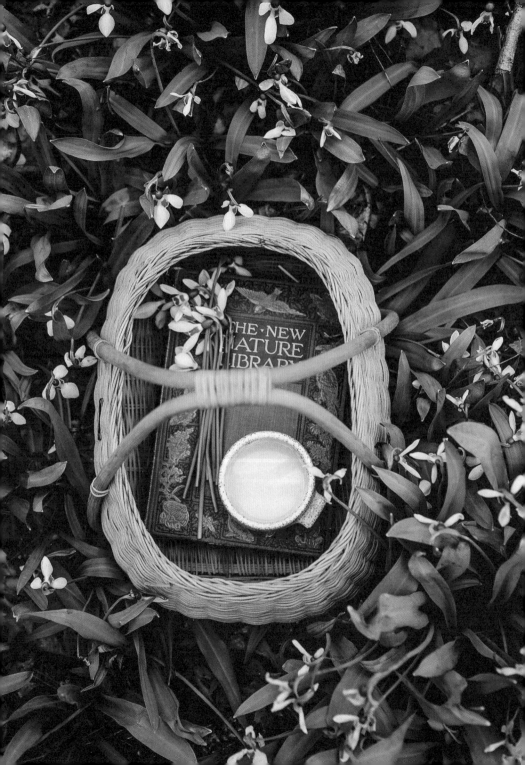

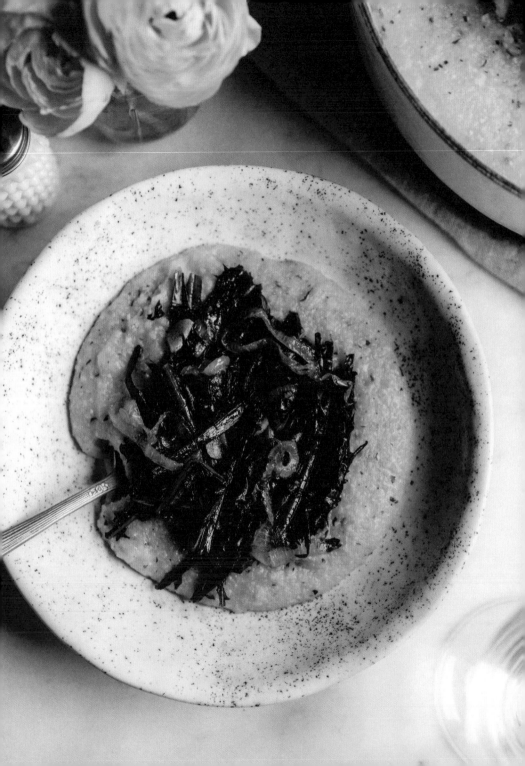

Mayi Moulen

Dandelion greens taste amazing served on top of polenta Haitian-style, known as mayi moulen. I remember when polenta became popular about ten or fifteen years ago. My mom was so confused when she ordered it in restaurants, because she knew it as a staple food from her childhood—not as a "trendy" food but as something simple that filled your belly when times were lean.

1 tablespoon extra-virgin olive oil

1 small onion, finely chopped

1 garlic clove, minced or thinly sliced

4½ cups filtered water

1 cup coarse yellow cornmeal

1 tablespoon finely chopped fresh flat-leaf parsley

½ teaspoon finely chopped fresh thyme

Salt and freshly ground black pepper

Makes 6 to 8 servings

Heat the oil in a heavy medium saucepan over medium heat and sauté the onion and garlic until translucent and golden, about 6 minutes. Add the filtered water and bring to a boil.

When the water boils, slowly pour in the cornmeal in a thin stream, stirring constantly. Add the parsley, thyme, and salt and pepper to taste. Stir constantly to avoid any lumps.

Lower the heat, simmer, and cook uncovered, stirring occasionally, until the cornmeal is tender with a soft but not runny consistency, 20 to 25 minutes. Adjust with more water or salt if necessary.

Dandelion Greens

This recipe explores the ability of spring greens to wake up your digestive system and detox your liver. These dandelion greens are an homage to the ancestral preparation of collard greens, done simply and with a little spice to make a lot out of a little. You can serve this over polenta (page 105) or as a side.

2 teaspoons salt

1 pound dandelion greens, torn into 4-inch pieces

2 tablespoons extra-virgin olive oil

1 tablespoon unsalted butter

½ onion, thinly sliced

¼ teaspoon crushed red pepper flakes

2 garlic cloves, minced

1 teaspoon paprika

Salt and freshly ground black pepper

Makes 4 servings

Bring a large pot of water and 1 teaspoon of the salt to a boil. Add greens and cook until tender, 3 to 4 minutes. Drain and rinse with cold water until chilled.

Heat the olive oil and butter in a large skillet over medium heat; when the butter melts, add the onion and red pepper flakes and cook until the onion is tender, about 5 minutes. Add the garlic and stir until fragrant, about 30 seconds more. Increase the heat to medium-high and add dandelion greens and paprika. Continue to stir until the liquid has evaporated, 3 to 4 minutes. Season with salt and black pepper.

Dandelion Greens and White Beans on Toast

Makes 6 to 8 servings

In a bowl of cold ice water and kosher salt, soak the dandelion greens. Heat the olive oil in a large Dutch oven over medium high heat. Add the onion, shallot, thyme, and flake salt. Cook for 6 minutes or so, until softened and translucent, stirring occasionally. Add the garlic and red pepper flakes and cook for 1 minute. Add the greens, beans, and stock, stir to combine and bring to a boil. Lower the heat and simmer until the liquid has reduced and thickened, about 8 minutes. Smash some of the beans with the back of a wooden spoon. Remove from the heat and stir in the lemon juice. Season to taste with salt. Serve over crusty toast.

3 cups chopped dandelion greens

2 tablespoons olive oil

1 medium onion, finely diced

1 shallot, minced

2 teaspoons fresh thyme

1 teaspoon kosher flake salt

3 garlic cloves, minced

¼ teaspoon crushed red pepper flakes

2 (14.5-ounce) cans white beans, rinsed and drained (I use Great Northern white beans)

1 cup vegetable stock

2 teaspoons lemon juice

Loaf of crusty bread, sliced and toasted

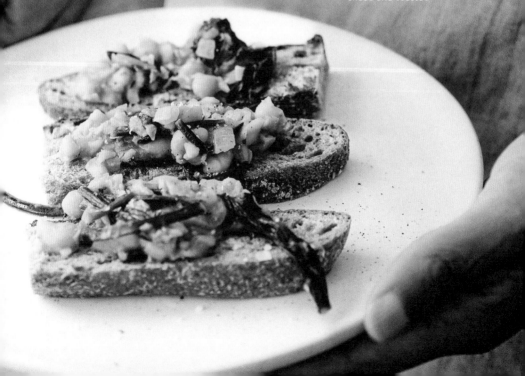

Garlic Mustard ALLIARIA PETIOLATA

*G*arlic mustard prefers to spread in shady areas as a groundcover. This biennial plant grows leaves in its first year and flowers that go to seed in its second year. Deemed a noxious weed and an invasive species brought by European settlers in the sixteenth century, their growth pattern can choke out native plant species. Pulling up the leaves in the first year and eating them, ensuring they do not flower and go to seed, is one way to eradicate them rather than spraying chemicals. They can nourish our bodies and we can help local ecosystems.

Garlic mustard greens are a nutritive wild green, containing vitamins A, B, and C along with potassium, calcium, magnesium, selenium, copper, iron, manganese, and omega-3 fatty acids. There are no concerns with overharvesting this plant, and we should all try to increase our usage of it, not only because it is invasive but also because it is tasty and so good for us. Include garlic mustard in sautéed greens, omelets, soups, mashed potatoes, and pesto—basically any place you might use garlic.

Plant family
Brassicaceae

Region
Native to Europe, western
and central Asia, North and
West Africa, the British Isles,
Pakistan, western China

Botanical description
Rounder leaves with scalloped
edges on first-year plants,
groundcover; flowers with
four small white petals and
triangular-shaped leaves the
following spring.

Herbal actions
Vermifuge, diaphoretic,
antiseptic

Energetics
Bitter

Flower essence
Focus your attention
and connect in alignment
with goals.

Gather
In spring for tender leaves,
reblooms in mild fall and
early winter

Grow
As this plant is an invasive
species, I would encourage
you to go out into the local
ecology to see if you can
forage and eat it; this will
assist the native species.

Preparations
Add to stir-fries, salads,
and pesto.

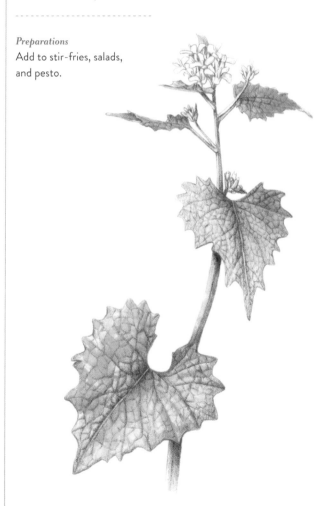

Garlic Mustard Pull-Apart Bread

Shortly after nettles emerge, I find garlic mustard hiding under the melting snow. Garlic mustard is an invasive species, and I will try and pull it up by its roots when I harvest it. Like its name portends, its pungent flavor is strikingly similar to garlic's. I love blending it up into a simple pesto, but I love this pull-apart bread even more.

Dough

2 teaspoons instant yeast

1 tablespoon honey or sugar

¾ cup milk

3 tablespoons unsalted butter, at room temperature

1 large egg

2⅓ cups (291g) all-purpose flour, plus more as needed

1 teaspoon salt

1 teaspoon garlic powder

2 tablespoons finely chopped fresh garlic mustard

Makes 1 loaf

Place the yeast and honey in a large mixing bowl. In a saucepan on medium heat, warm the milk on the stove until warm to touch, about 110°F (43°C). Pour the warm milk on top of yeast/honey mixture. Whisk gently to combine, then loosely cover with a clean kitchen towel and allow it to sit for 5 to 10 minutes, until the mixture is frothy.

Add the butter, egg, flour, salt, garlic powder, and garlic mustard to the milk/yeast/honey mixture and blend. The dough will be soft. Transfer to a lightly floured work surface. Using lightly floured hands, knead the dough for 1 minute. If the dough is too sticky to handle, add up to 3 more tablespoons flour, but you want a very soft dough. Shape the dough into a ball.

Place the dough in an oiled bowl and cover with a kitchen towel. Place in a slightly warm environment to rise until doubled in size for 1 to 1½ hours.

As the dough rises, grease a 9 × 5-inch loaf pan and prepare the filling. In a medium bowl, mix the softened butter, garlic mustard, rosemary, garlic, and salt together with a fork. Cover it tightly and set aside at room temperature until ready to use (keeping it at room temperature makes it easier to spread).

Herbed Butter Filling

4 tablespoons unsalted
butter, at room temperature

1 tablespoon finely chopped
fresh garlic mustard

1 tablespoon finely chopped
fresh rosemary, or
2 teaspoons dried

2 garlic cloves, minced,
or ½ teaspoon garlic powder

¼ teaspoon salt

Melted butter (optional)

Flaky or coarse sea salt,
for sprinkling

Place dough on a lightly floured work surface. Divide it into 12 equal pieces, about 3 tablespoons each, and shape them into balls. With lightly floured hands, flatten each into a disk about 4 inches in diameter. Spread 1 teaspoon of the herbed butter onto each. Fold each disk in half and line them in prepared baking pan, round side up.

Cover the pan with a kitchen towel and put in a warm spot to rise for 40 to 50 minutes. The dough should be puffy and double in size.

Preheat the oven to 350°F. Uncover the pan and bake until the bread is golden brown, about 50 minutes. Turn down the temperature to 325°F and cover with foil if the top is browning too quickly. Remove from the oven and place the pan on a wire rack. If desired, brush with melted butter for topping and sprinkle with sea salt. Cool the bread in the pan for 10 minutes, then remove from the pan and serve warm.

Cover and store leftovers at room temperature for up to 2 days or in the refrigerator for up to 1 week.

Lilac SYRINGA VULGARIS

Lilac is a signature of Midwestern spring ushering in a spirit of renewal. Found in vacant lots, roadsides, woodlands, and around abandoned homesteads, lilacs are fleeting and finite, blooming for a couple weeks in spring. On the wave of climate chaos, it has started to bloom again in the late fall. The four-petaled flowers are found in a range from white to deep purple, with a pale purple being the most popular. This flowering shrub is a member of the olive family and originated in the Balkans; immigrants brought the shrub to plant in the gardens in northern Europe, introducing it into English gardens in the sixteenth century and to the United States upon the heels of colonization in the eighteenth century.

The floral scent of lilac is intoxicating but truly hard to capture and preserve. While many people enjoy lilacs as fresh-cut flowers on their tables, lilacs also have health benefits and powerful energetics that have been used in folk medicine since the Middle Ages. Along with being aromatic, lilac's bitter and astringent nature helps lower fever and improve digestion. In folk medicine, it was commonly used to treat parasitic and intestinal worms. Preserved in oil and used on the skin, it soothes inflamed and irritated skin and can treat sunburns and rashes.

Make sure to use only the flowers, as the bark can be toxic. Sprinkle flowers into baked goods and salads, or preserve them in honey or sugar.

CAUTION: Bark can be toxic. Exercise caution if consuming lilacs in addition to blood-thinning medications.

You can also make lilac water to sip or spritz on the face as an uplifting spring delight by adding a handful of fresh lilac blooms to a pint of filtered water, refrigerated for 4 to 8 hours. Strain and sip.

Plant family
Oleaceae

Other names
Common lilac, lila in Bosnia and Haitian Creole

Region
Originated in southeastern Europe and the Balkans, now cultivated worldwide

Botanical description
Deciduous shrub, new shoots are green, while old growth is gray. Bark is rough and gray. Simple, opposite leaves, oval and pinnate. Aromatic tubular flowers in spring range in color from lavender to white; four united petals and four united sepals arranged in dense conical shape.

Herbal actions
Astringent

Energetics
Bitter, acrid

Flower essence
We can confront painful memories and trauma, but we also need to hold space for joy and new purpose.

Gather
In May, collect dry flowers in the morning or evening, selecting the heads with fresh and newly opened blossoms (steer clear of brown blooms)

Grow
Prefers neutral, well-drained soils in full sun; grows as a large shrub or small tree

Preparations
Preserved in sugar, water, jelly, lemonade, honey, syrups, and wine

Lilac Syrup

I love preserving the floral aromas and medicinal qualities of flowers in syrups. Some of my favorite spring floral syrups include violet, honeysuckle, rose, and this lilac syrup recipe.

Syrups can be mixed into drinks and baked goods for flavoring and have been used medicinally as well. Sugar is commonly used in syrups and acts as a preservative, whereas syrups made with honey are more prone to spoilage. Syrups made with honey should be refrigerated.

1 cup sugar or honey

2 or 3 blueberries or blackberries to enhance the color (optional)

2 cups packed lilac florets, flowers only, green parts removed (see Note)

1 teaspoon lemon juice

Makes 16 ounces or 2 cups

In a small saucepan over medium heat, combine the sweetener, blueberries if using, and 2 cups water and cook until the sweetener has dissolved. Remove the saucepan from the heat and let the mixture cool. Add the unrinsed blooms to a jar, pour the cooled syrup mixture over the blooms, stir in the lemon juice, and cover with a lid. Put the jar in the refrigerator and steep for 24 to 48 hours; begin testing after 24 hours for your desired flavor. Strain and pour into a sterilized jar. This will keep for 2 months in the refrigerator.

Add 2 to 4 tablespoons to sparkling water for a refreshing spring soda. As you sip, meditate on memories, moments, and little joys that rejuvenate your spirit.

NOTE
Do not rinse the florets or they can lose their delicate flavor.

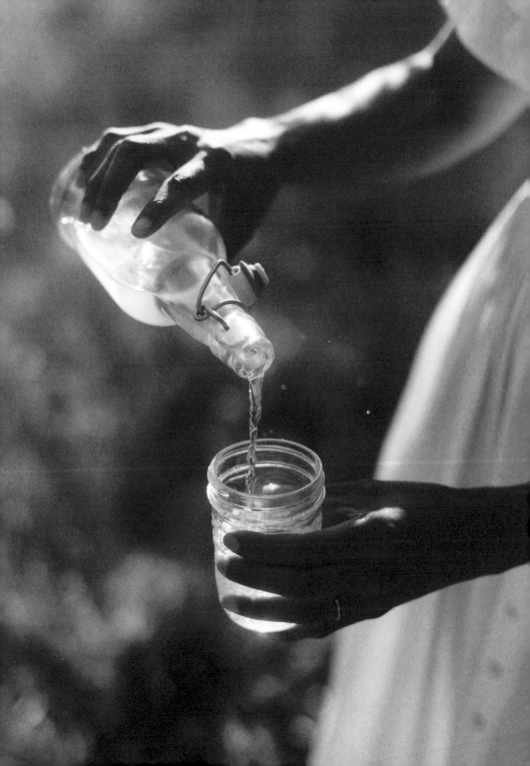

Lilac Lemonade Ice Pops

Lilac lemonade Ice Pops provide instant gratification and are a huge hit in our home in late spring. The flavor is light, floral, and refreshing, with a hint of pucker from the lemons. The sour taste is wonderful at cooling the body, especially when late spring is almost eighty degrees here in the Midwest and we all want something refreshing.

1 cup lemon juice
(4 to 6 lemons)

1 cup packed lilac flowers, green parts removed

¾ to 1 cup honey

Makes 6 ice pops

Strain the lemon juice and set aside.

Separate lilac flowers from any green parts. Combine the lilacs and 2 cups water in a small saucepan over medium heat and bring to a simmer. Remove the pan from heat, cover, and set aside for 15 to 20 minutes.

Strain lilac infusion into a bowl and stir in the honey to taste until dissolved. Add the lemon juice to the lilac syrup.

Pour the lilac lemonade into ice-pop molds according to the manufacturer's directions (leave a tiny 1 to 2 mm clearance at the top for expansion). Sprinkle lilac flowers on top, insert sticks into the mixture, and freeze until solid, 4 to 8 hours.

Nettle URTICA DIOICA

A s you walk along a patch of prairie, near a creek or at the woods' edge, growing in damp nitrogen-rich soils, nettle's sting may pull you in, bringing your attention to its presence. You may need to make friends. Nettles are a nutritive plant that has been gathered for thousands of years as a prized food and friend. Found across the world in temperate climates, nettle is fortifying. Nettles sting for a reason: protection. But don't be deterred by the sting; I often find it's lessened the more I work with the plant. You can wear gloves to pick and process it, but I often harvest nettles bare hands by holding the underside, clipping the stem, and gently placing it in my basket. Traditionally, nettle stings were purposefully used topically to reduce inflammation and arthritis. Growing nettle in your garden can reduce pest infestation for other plants, as nettles attract beneficial insects, including predatory insects and native bees.

Drying, cooking, or adding them to hot water rids the nettles of their sting, and from there, their uses are endless. Nettles are rich in iron and contain vitamins A, B complex, and C, zinc, magnesium, calcium, and potassium, all nutrients that act to build our bodies and our immune systems. Nettle infusions can help with the sluggish symptoms of premenstrual syndrome (PMS). Nettles' antihistamine properties are a wonderful treatment for hay fever, in the form of tincture or tea. Nettle seeds in small doses support the adrenal system.

Nettles are a detoxifying spring tonic, cleansing and clearing and nourishing our systems after a long winter and driving out unwanted energies. They are found in nitrogen-rich soils such as the woods, fields, and alongside rivers. I use the tender spring greens in frittatas and pesto, and gather nettles later in the spring and into early summer to dry for winter infusions. Nettles are not for everyone—check with your doctor if you're diabetic, as they can modify glucose regulation.

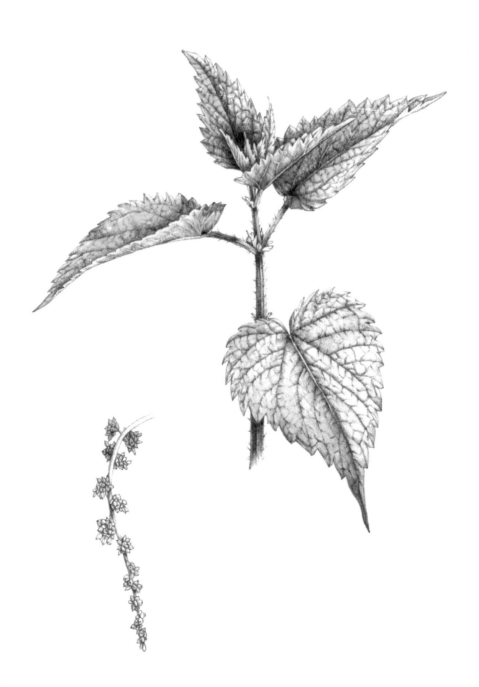

Plant family
Urticaceae

Other names
Common nettle, stinging nettle

Region
USDA Plant Hardiness Zones 3 to 10. Found throughout temperate regions worldwide, though mainly in the Northern Hemisphere, in nitrogen-rich soils, woodlands, and prairies.

Botanical description
Serrated, heart-shaped leaves with stinging hairs, opposite leaves with pointed tips. Hairy, square stems with spines, purple to green tops in the spring.

Herbal actions
Antihistamine, anti-inflammatory, alterative, astringent, diuretic, kidney tonic, nutritive

Energetics
Cooling and drying

Flower essence
It helps you identify and change toxic behaviors, patterns, and relationships, imbuing you with clarity, flexibility, and the strength to change.

Gather
The most succulent young leaves in the spring, can harvest into the summer before the plant flowers and goes to seed. Gather seeds by shaking them from a plant into a jar in the fall for winter/spring planting. Refrain from gathering nettles along roadsides or locations with contaminated soils.

Grow
Nettle can be grown from seed or divided from a patch in late fall. It prefers moist soils, in full sun to partial shade, 80 to 90 days to maturity. The small seeds require light for germination. Can be raked or pressed lightly into the soil in early spring, ¼ inch deep, or sown indoors in late winter and planted as soon as the ground can be worked.

Body systems affinities
Urinary tract, immune system, nervous and circulatory system

Preparations
Cooked in pesto, soups, and eggs; dried in infusions and teas, tinctures, infused vinegars; substitute for spinach in food recipes

Rustic Nettle Tart

*My dear friend Hannah helped us find our cottage home, and
she left a tart in our refrigerator on moving day. It felt like
such a gift of friendship and nourishment, and every time I eat
this tart, I feel deeply cherished, satisfied, and cared for.*

*Makes
4 to 6
servings*

Preheat the oven to 425°F.

To prepare the pastry, whisk together the flour
and 1 teaspoon of the salt in a medium bowl. With a
fork or spatula, stir in the olive oil and ⅓ cup of the milk until
well blended. This pastry is rustic and will be crumbly; use your
hands to press it evenly into a 9-inch pie pan or tart pan with
a removable bottom. Press the pastry evenly up the sides and
prick the bottom all over with a fork.

Bake the shell for 10 to 15 minutes, until golden brown.
Meanwhile in a large cast-iron skillet, if using bacon, cook
chopped bacon over medium-high heat until crispy. Reserve
the cooking grease or add olive oil over medium heat and
sauté the red onion until tender. Add the chopped nettles and
sauté until wilted. Stir in the garlic, thyme, pepper, and the
remaining ¼ teaspoon salt. Continue to cook over medium-low
heat until well softened, stirring occasionally. Remove from
the heat.

In a large bowl combine the eggs, the remaining ⅓ cup milk,
and 1 cup of the Parmesan (if using).

Stir in the nettle mixture, then scrape the mixture into the
prepared tart shell. Sprinkle the remaining ¼ cup Parmesan (if
using) on top of the tart before placing it in the oven. Reduce
the oven temperature to 375°F and bake until the filling is
firm, 25 to 35 minutes.

1¾ cups all-purpose flour
(or gluten-free flour)

1¼ teaspoons kosher salt

½ cup plus 2 tablespoons
extra-virgin olive oil

⅔ cup milk, my preference
is nondairy milk

¼ cup chopped bacon
(optional)

1 small red onion, finely diced

¾ pound fresh nettles,
leaves and tops chopped

2 garlic cloves, finely diced

1 teaspoon
freshly chopped thyme

½ teaspoon
freshly cracked pepper

5 large eggs

1 cup plus ¼ cup grated
Parmesan cheese (optional)

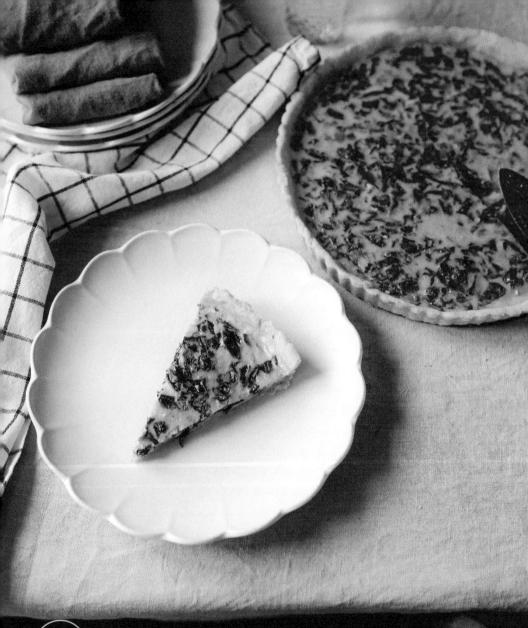

NOTE

I love preserving nettles. Fill a large saucepan with water and bring to a boil. Add 10 cups washed nettles and let boil for 30 seconds, until bright green. Remove the nettles with a slotted spoon and plunge them in an ice bath, reserving the cooking water. Add the nettles and ¼ cup of the reserved water to a blender. Puree until smooth; you can add up to another quarter cup of the cooking liquid as necessary for a smooth mixture. Pour the nettle puree into an ice cube tray, dividing it evenly, and freeze overnight. Remove the cubes and place in a freezer-safe storage bag or jar.

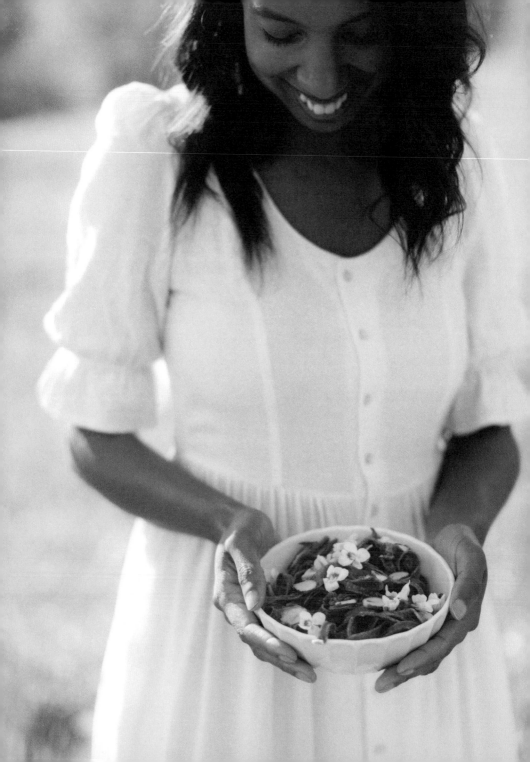

Nettle Pasta

Nettle pasta is just one of many ways to incorporate nettles into your diet. Griffin will eat a whole bowl of fresh nettle pasta simply with melted butter, salt, and pepper.

2 cups packed
stinging nettle leaves

1 large whole egg plus 3 yolks

1½ cups all-purpose flour
(or substitute all-purpose
gluten-free flour), plus more
for dusting

Splash of olive oil

Serves 4

Bring a medium pot of water to a boil. Prepare a bowl of ice water.

When the water comes to a boil, add the nettles using tongs. Blanch the nettles for 1 minute, then remove them using a slotted spoon and place them in the prepared ice bath to stop the cooking. Once cool, they are safe to handle with your hands. Drain them and squeeze out any remaining water. Coarsely chop the nettles and add them to a food processor or blender, along with the whole egg and the yolks. Pulse several times to combine well.

Add flour and pulse or blend until the mixture pulls away from the sides. Alternatively, you can mound the flour on a work surface and add the nettle-egg mixture to the center, kneading it for 5 to 8 minutes, until the dough comes together and is no longer sticky. Shape the dough into a disk shape, wrap in plastic, and refrigerate for 1 hour. Use a pasta maker, following the manufacturer's instructions, or if making by hand, use your hands to roll out the pasta to ⅛ inch thick and use a sharp knife to cut into your preferred shape. Dust the pasta lightly with flour and swirl into a nest on parchment paper or hang to dry.

To prepare the pasta, bring a large pot of water to a boil and add the pasta and a splash of olive oil. Remove pasta when it floats to the surface. You can use this recipe to make raviolis as well.

Oven–Roasted Risotto with Nettle Pesto

Oven-roasted risotto is one of our family favorites, Magnolia in particular. This recipe is a simple weeknight comfort food.

Makes 4 to 6 servings

Preheat the oven to 350°F. Heat 2 tablespoons of the olive oil in a large Dutch oven over medium heat. Add the onions and cook, stirring, until onions are soft. Stir in the rice and salt and pepper to taste and cook until the grains are translucent, about 5 minutes.

Add the wine and simmer until it evaporates. Add 2 cups of the broth, bring to a simmer, cover, and place in the oven. Cook until the liquid is mostly absorbed, about 15 minutes. Remove from oven, stir in the pesto, and, if desired, top with toasted walnuts and grated Parmesan cheese.

4 tablespoons extra-virgin olive oil

1 small white onion

1 cup arborio rice

Salt and freshly ground black pepper

½ cup dry white wine

2 cups broth or water

2 cups of Nettle Pesto

¼ cup toasted walnuts and grated Parmesan cheese, for topping (optional)

Nettle Pesto

In a food processor, pulse the pepitas and garlic until the pepitas are ground. Add the salt and pepper and pulse again to mix.

Add the blanched nettles and lemon juice. With the food processor running, drizzle in the olive oil and process until combined. Season to taste.

½ cup pepitas

1 small garlic clove

Heaping ¼ teaspoon sea salt

Freshly ground black pepper

4 packed cups fresh nettles, blanched (see page 123)

2 tablespoons lemon juice

½ cup extra-virgin olive oil

Nettle Seasoning

This savory blend is delicious sprinkled on eggs, popcorn, and roasted vegetables. It combines flavor and herbal nutrition in one spoonful.

¼ cup white sesame seeds

1 tablespoon seaweed, such as dulse, kelp, or nori

1 tablespoon dried nettle

1 tablespoon sage

1 tablespoon ground sumac

1 tablespoon kosher sea salt

Makes 8 servings

Place sesame seeds on the bottom of a frying pan, covering the entire bottom (I like to use my cast-iron pan). Heat the seeds over medium heat until lightly fragrant. Remove the seeds before they toast.

Combine the seaweed, dried nettle, sage, and sumac in a mortar and pestle and grind for about 5 minutes. You can also lightly pulse them in a food processor but be careful that it doesn't turn into a paste. Combine the ground seaweed and herbs, salt, and sesame seeds and store in an airtight jar for up to 2 weeks. Sprinkle the mixture lavishly on your favorite foods, like Roasted Squash (page 270) or popcorn.

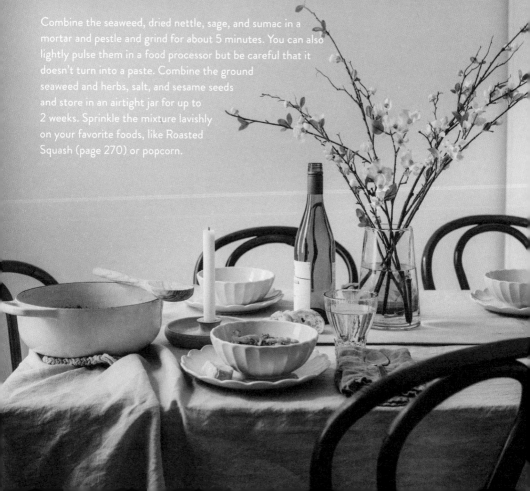

Spring Minestrone

Makes 8 servings

¼ cup extra-virgin olive oil

1 large yellow onion, finely diced

1 teaspoon ground coriander

1 teaspoon fennel seeds, ground

½ teaspoon whole black peppercorns

4 garlic cloves, thinly sliced

½ teaspoon crushed red pepper flakes

2 large leeks, white and pale green parts only, tough outer layers removed, sliced into ½-inch-thick rounds

1 fennel bulb, halved lengthwise, fronds coarsely chopped for garnish

1 bay leaf

6 cups herbal broth or bone broth

Zest and juice from 1 lemon

1 (15.5-ounce) can white cannellini beans, rinsed and drained

2 cups sugar snap peas or peas (shelled fresh or thawed frozen)

Kosher salt

2 cups fresh nettle leaves, stems removed, roughly chopped

1 tablespoon white miso

Freshly ground black pepper

¼ cup chopped fresh parsley

Grated pecorino cheese (optional)

Heat the olive oil, the onion, the ground spices, and the peppercorns in a large Dutch oven over medium heat, stirring often, until the onion is softened, about 5 minutes. Add the garlic and cook for 2 minutes. Add red pepper flakes, leeks, fennel bulb, and bay leaf and cook, stirring occasionally, for 5 minutes, or until softened.

Pour the broth into the Dutch oven, increase the heat to medium-high, and bring to a simmer, cooking until the broth is fragrant, about 30 minutes. Add the lemon zest and juice, salt to taste, beans, and sugar snap peas (the vegetables will shrink as they cook). Lower the heat to medium. Simmer, stirring occasionally, until the leeks, fennel, and sugar snap peas are fork-tender, about 5 minutes. Add the chopped nettle, shelled peas, fennel fronds, and miso and cook, stirring constantly, just until the nettle is wilted, about 30 seconds; season with more salt and some freshly ground black pepper to taste.

Ladle the soup into bowls and top with chopped parsley and grated pecorino cheese, if desired. The soup can be made a day ahead; transfer the soup or any leftovers to an airtight container and chill. Reheat before serving.

A Tutorial on Flower Essences

For me, the first flower essences of spring are magical. After waiting all winter long, flowers—the portals to energetic healing—have arrived. It is potent medicine to just sit and be with the energy of a flower, dancing in the breeze and existing as the highest manifestation of its life-form. Flower essences capture the vibrational medicine of a flower in water through the sun's rays and preserve it with alcohol. Flower essences work on the subtle layers of the energy body to help heal and clear psychological and emotional blockages.

Take a couple of deep, cleansing breaths and gather your materials with intention and an open heart. You will need water, a glass bowl, and a pair of scissors. Find a flower that has come to you, perhaps while you were exploring or maybe in a dream. That flower may want to work with you. Intention and connection are the most important aspects of crafting a flower essence.

Ask permission before cutting each flower, paying attention for a sign. Maybe a slight breeze causes the plant to nod, or a bee might land nearby.

Make sure the flowers or blooms you are using are not sprayed with pesticides, herbicides, or fungicides for your own health and well-being. Cut the flower or multiple flowers into the bowl of water. Use your intuition to know how many blooms your essence needs. Then place the bowl in full sunlight for 3 to 5 hours to imprint the vibration of the flower onto the water. I have also made a flower essence at night under a full moon.

When your essence is ready, strain out the flowers, pouring the water and blooms through a funnel lined with cheesecloth into a bottle or jar. Place the blooms you've used back on the earth with gratitude.

Preserve this original mother essence with 50/50 alcohol. Traditionally, brandy is used, and I often use organic vodka. Apple cider vinegar can also be used; in which case, the essence should be refrigerated for longevity.

Label your flower essence with the name of the flower, date, and location where it was gathered, and any specific details you may want to remember later. I often record the moon phase and what sign the moon is in. This is now your preserved mother essence.

A stock bottle is made from 1 to 7 drops of the mother essence in a 50/50 solution of water and alcohol.

A dosage bottle is made with 1 to 7 drops of the stock essence in a 50/50 solution of water and alcohol. Dosage bottles are great for making blends of flower essences using between 1 and 7 drops of up to six different flowers in a blend.

The stock bottle works on the acute physical symptoms and emotional realm, and a dosage bottle works on the most subtle energies.

How to Use Your Flower Essence

Take 2 to 4 drops up to four times a day from the stock and dosage bottles. You can place them directly on your tongue, massage acupressure points on the body, in your drinking water, or into a healing bath. Potency is increased not by taking more drops at a time but instead with consistent use.

Plantain Plantago spp.

*P*lantain grows where our feet carry us. Commonly referred to as white man's footsteps, they are found where colonization has taken them, can withstand heavy foot traffic, and are spread through soil disturbance and compaction. In lawns, on footpaths, and in grasslands, plantain is an all-around ally for soothing the skin, especially in the late spring and summer months. Broadleaf plantain can be used much like a bandage over a wound or chewed up into a spit poultice for a bee sting. Its young leaves contain vitamins A, C, and K and are edible either raw in a salad or cooked and added to your wild greens repertoire, as it has calcium and mucilage.

Plantain has numerous medicinal properties and can be applied to the skin to soothe inflammation, sores, bug bites, stings, and rashes. Plantain also acts as a vulnerary for intestinal membranes and can soothe inflammation in the gut lining. Although carried by colonization, it has become naturalized and is a potent remedy packaged in a common weed—a plant stepped on and trampled, but still resilient and helpful.

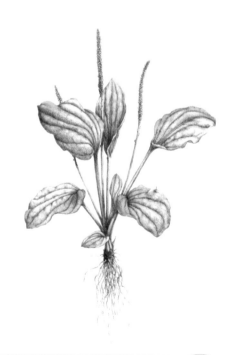

Plant family
Plantaginaceae

Other names
Englishman's foot, white man's footsteps

Region
Introduced from Eurasia, plaintain is now found throughout Europe, North Africa, north and central Asia, and most temperate climates (including North America) and some tropical areas.

Botanical description
Low green rosette with basal leaves, parallel leaf veins, small green flowers on a slender stalk

Herbal actions
Antibacterial, anti-inflammatory, antiviral, astringent, demulcent, vulnerary

Energetics
Cooling

Flower essence
Helps release bitterness and mental blocks

Gather
Leaves any time in the season before the plant flowers, late spring to early fall; seeds from midsummer to late fall

Body systems affinities
Digestive and skin

Preparations
Infused oil, eaten raw, seeds used as a thickening agent, poultice

Violet VIOLA SPP.

Violets are an early perennial spring plant, a groundcover that spreads its roots underground. It displays a soft and humble flower growing underfoot in moist and shaded areas of gardens and woodlands. For violet, the doctrine of signatures is strong; as indicated by its heart-shaped leaves, it works on the heart, lungs, and circulatory system. Violet reminds us of the softness that can be reached when we work with the heart.

Violet's nature is cooling and soothing; it quenches heat, both physically and emotionally, easing fevers and hives. The Cherokee used violet's soothing nature as a remedy for coughs, colds, and respiratory infections. Violet is an expectorant, demulcent, alterative, anti-inflammatory, and diuretic. A fully edible plant, you can use violet leaves in oils, infuse violet flowers and leaves in wine, and add flowers in baked goods.

Plant family
Violaceae

Common name
Pansy

Region
Most species are found in temperate climates in the Northern Hemisphere, but some species are found worldwide. There are more than six hundred species of violets (Elpel, 2013).

Botanical description
Heart-shaped, scalloped leaves. Drooping flowers of white to violet with five petals.

Gather
Leaves and flowers in the spring and fall.

Herbal actions
Expectorant, demulcent, alterative, anti-inflammatory, diuretic

Energetics
Cooling and drying

Flower essence
Calming, offers connection; sharing with others while remaining true to oneself; overcoming shyness

Preparations
Violet leaf infused oil, edible in salads, floral ice cubes, syrups, sugared violets

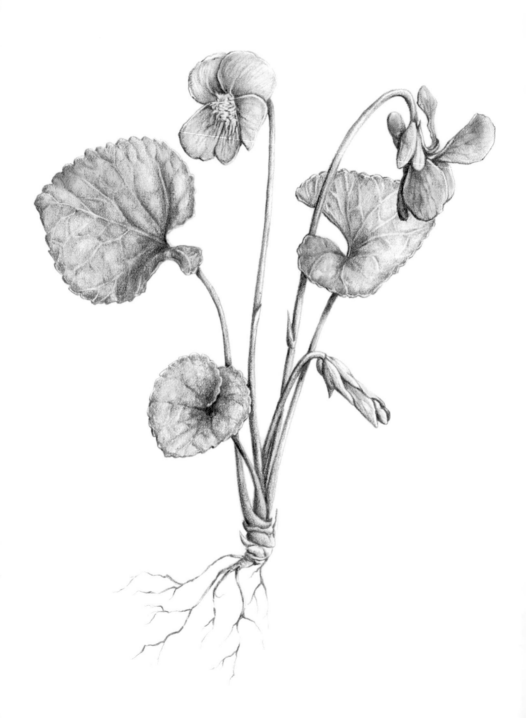

Violet Lemonade

Violets are a welcome sight in spring. I love to collect them with the children in our garden and the woods. This recipe is so fun because the addition of the lemon juice turns this lemonade into a bright shade of violet!

1 cup packed fresh purple violets

3 cups filtered water

2 tablespoons raw honey

4 to 6 lemons, halved and juiced

Frozen blueberries, for serving

Makes 4 servings

Carefully rinse the violets and combine them with the filtered water in a saucepan, bring to a boil over medium heat, then cover, turn down the heat, and simmer for 10 to 15 minutes, until the infusion turns blue. Remove from the heat and let cool for 5 minutes. Strain this violet infusion through a mesh sieve into a jar—it should be blue! Add the honey. Stir or cover tightly with a lid and shake to dissolve the honey. Let cool. Add fresh squeezed lemon juice and mix again. This should turn your violet lemonade pink! Top off with frozen blueberries and serve.

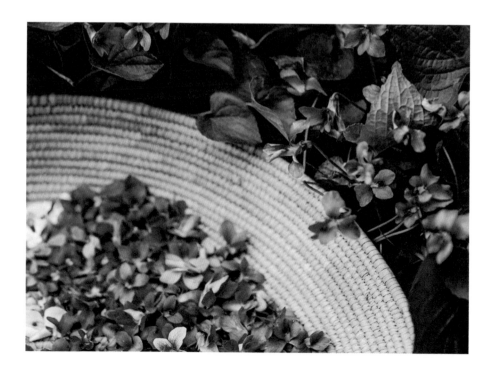

Violet Leaf Infused Oil

Makes 1 pint jar

Collect a handful or more of violet's heart-shaped leaves and wilt them on a screen or in a basket for 24 hours.

Fill a pint-size jar with dried violet leaves. Cover with your chosen carrier oil and seal with lid. Store in a dark place for 4 to 6 weeks, shaking occasionally. Strain through cheesecloth and mesh sieve into a sterilized glass jar, seal tightly, and label with the date, plant name, and oil used and store it in a cool dark place.

Use this cooling oil for inflamed skin conditions (including eczema), sunburn, inflammation, rashes, and hives. It is also a wonderful addition to a breast massage and lymphatic oil with red clover.

Bug–bite Oil

Made with violet-infused oil, plantain oil, and lavender essential oil, this is a cooling oil for heat conditions on the skin and bug bites in the summer.

4 ounces violet infused oil

4 ounces plantain infused oil

15 drops lavender essential oil

Makes 8 ounces

Combine the infused oils in a bowl and add essential oil. Stir well, pour oil into an amber bottle or an amber bottle with a roller ball lid for easy application to irritated skin.

To apply, rub a small amount onto bug bite or irritated skin with a clean hand two or three times a day.

Spiritual Cleansing Bath for the Full Flower Moon

Herbal baths are an important part of Haitian culture (Volpato, 2009), seen as a physical representation of emotional, magical, physical, and spiritual needs. It's important to choose herbs that work with your emotional states to help cleanse the body, mind, and spirit of residue. You can gather flowers from the garden or your walk, making sure the flowers are not sprayed with pesticides, herbicides, or fungicides.

To prepare an herbal bath tea, place your herbs in a French press filled with boiling water. Let steep for 30 minutes. While the tea steeps, shower yourself, dry brush or scrub your body with a washcloth, loofah, or salt scrub, cleansing the skin and purifying the body. This aids in shedding our old skins and opening the body to receive the healing medicine floral bath. Clean the tub and prepare your bath by running warm to hot water, as desired. Add ¼ cup Epsom salts and 2 tablespoons magnesium flakes to the tub, pour in the herbal bath tea, and float fresh flowers. Carefully climb into the water and allow your body, mind, and spirit to be infused with the uplifting and nourishing spirit of the plants and enjoy. A foot bath works as well to cleanse and ground your energy.

SUGGESTED PLANTS: Violets, yarrow, hollyhocks, rose petals, chamomile.

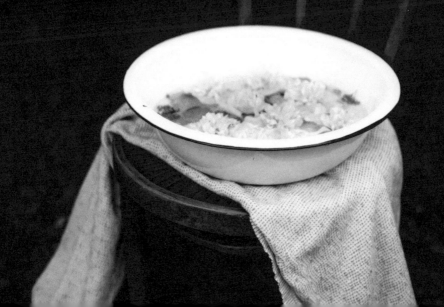

Summer

Seasonal Wisdom

Exhalation, light, alive, verdant,
capture the energy from the sun,
production, courage, will, growth,
the maiden, blooming, midday,
passion, energy

Summer solstice
June 22

Astrology of summer
Cancer (cardinal water),
Leo (fixed fire), Virgo (mutable earth)

Energetics of summer
Hot, becoming dry

Element
Fire

Chakra
Solar plexus and heart

Direction
South

Of
Flower
and Fruit

:

Full Moon

:

Adolescence

:

Growth
and Abundance

:

South

*S*ummer is a time of celebration. We gather, we play, we learn, we explore, we look beyond ourselves. Yang energy is rising; there is an outward manifestation of the dreams that were born in our hearts in late winter and early spring. We begin to see the fruits of our hard work and dreaming. The plants are at their peak, and we seek a relationship with the natural world. The weeds are also growing in this season. It is time to harness our discernment and weed out what isn't working. What do we want growing in our literal and metaphorical gardens?

Roses in our garden bloom in late May or early June. Strawberries ripen underfoot as the full Strawberry Moon rises in the summer skies. Elderflower blooms as the solstice approaches, and sweetness drips from the air. Our hearts beam wide open when the sun is at its strongest. We embody the sun's luminosity and joy. There is a euphoria about this season of blooms. Steep summer sun teas on the back porch. Harvest and hang clovers, yarrow, rose petals, and lemon balm for winter tea. Milkweed feeds the bees and the monarchs. Herbs of the sun make their appearance—calendula, St. John's wort, California poppy—and portend the chakras of summer, the solar plexus and heart. Currants and black raspberries ripen with the sun's rays, warm berries ready to be plucked and gathered.

Heat sets in. We seek cooling remedies for our minds and our bodies and refuge at the water's edge. Sour flavors are cooling, nervines can help with irritation and stress. Herbal lemonades and summer shrubs infused with elderflower, lemon balm, lavender, rose, and linden are tasty and provide relief.

In late August, as oppressive summer heat gives way to dry autumn air, we understand how to care for our bodies with the season. It's time to preserve seasonal foods: pickles, jams, ripe and juicy strawberries. Queen Anne's lace opens its umbels and sways in the prairies at sunset. Elder's flowers turn to berries.

As we drive home, goldenrod appears overnight in the rolling prairies. Could it be? The old adage says when goldenrod appears, first frost is six weeks away. The early apples begin to fill out. I make tinctures of fresh yarrow, St. John's wort, lemon balm, and holy basil while the plants are at their peak. I tuck herbs dried earlier in the seasons into glass jars. Harvest sumac, goldenrod, and apples at the full Sturgeon Moon. Celebration in community is the outward expression of energy, but our thoughts turn inward to preparation for the next season.

Calendula CALENDULA OFFICINALIS

Calendula, a self-sowing annual, reseeds itself in my garden each year. A member of the Asteraceae family, calendula is considered an herb of the sun, holding the warmth in its energy. In its native habitat, it is found on roadsides and in abandoned prairies. Warming and drying, calendula is a demulcent. A vulnerary herb, it works on the skin, inside and out, to regenerate, to heal and is a powerful wound- and tissue-healing plant. Collect flowers after the morning dew has dried. You can harvest just the flowering top or cut the flowers, leaves, and stems.

Calendula works on the solar plexus center of the body, strengthening the will, the spirit, and the resolve. Its bitter taste hints at its use for stimulating digestion, and it can soothe inflammation of the digestive tract, ulcers, and gastric reflux. I love adding calendula blooms to my winter broths and teas. Infused in oil or in a tincture, calendula's antimicrobial, antibiotic, and anti-inflammatory properties make it beneficial for cuts, burns, bites, rashes, sunburns, and diaper rash.

Calendula also works on the lymphatic system, stimulating circulation and removing toxins from the lymph and lymph nodes. Healthy lymph encourages a healthy immune system. Sprinkle calendula petals in salads, cookies, cakes, and soups. The petals are used in yellow dye and food coloring. It is a sunny ally that is easy to grow in the garden and a key companion plant. Easily tucked between food crops, calendula attracts beneficial pollinators and insects such as ladybugs, and its resinous blooms deter pests and act as a trap. Collect seeds after the seed heads turn from green to brown, lay them flat to dry, then save them in a jar or seed envelope for many years.

CAUTION: Although there are very few safety concerns with calendula, it should not be used during early pregnancy and may cause allergic reactions for those sensitive to other Asteraceae family members (like ragweed).

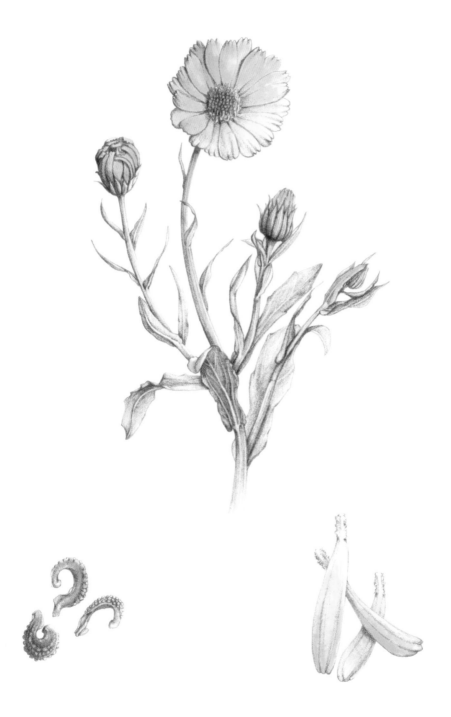

Plant family
Asteraceae

- -

Other names
Marigold, pot marigold,
garden marigold

- -

Region
Native to North Africa, Iran,
Egypt, the Mediterranean
region and southern Europe,
now widely distributed in
temperate regions

- -

Botanical description
Reaches 2 feet in height, with
waxy, smooth stems;
alternate, oblong, hairy, and
simple leaves; large, resinous
flower heads, ranging from
bright orange to bronze,
composed of many tiny
flowers in a floral disk with ray
florets attached to the center.

- -

Herbal actions
Anti-inflammatory,
antimicrobial, antifungal,
antispasmodic, hemostatic,
lymphatic, vulnerary,
astringent

Energetics
Warming, drying

- -

Flower essence
Cultivating receptivity in
human relationships—how to
listen more deeply with
empathy for others

- -

Parts used
Flowers and leaves

- -

Gather
Harvest flowers continually
from early summer through
late fall, in the morning when
the resin is sticky and dry.

- -

Grow
USDA Hardiness Zones 2–11
(cultivated in gardens). Seeds
can be sown directly in the
garden or started indoors 6 to
8 weeks before your region's
last frost. Tuck seeds ¼ to
½ inch deep into the soil;
calendula seeds require
darkness to germinate. Once
they germinate, plant them in
the garden after the last frost.
Pinch the first bud to
encourage more bushy plants.

Collect the blooms; pinching
the flowers off the stem (also
known as deadheading) will
encourage more blooms all
season long. For continuous
blooms, sow seeds every 3 to
4 weeks all season until
1 month before the first frost
in the fall.

- -

Preparations
Flowers petals are edible; use
also in infused oil, salves,
baths, poultices, soaks,
vinegars, tinctures, tea,
broths, and soups. Eat young
leaves raw in salads.

Catnip NEPETA CATARIA

*L*ong associated with a hypnotic effect in cats, the flowering mint catnip is a common folk remedy for digestive woes, nervousness, and fevers. The compound nepetalactone causes the reaction in some cats, but it also repels unwanted insects, like Japanese beetles, aphids, and squash bugs. A plant for more than cats, catnip in the garden is a friend to bees and hummingbirds alike, attracting beneficial pollinators to the garden. Catnip is a member of the Lamiaceae, or mint, family. A common remedy of enslaved Africans and widely used in Indigenous American medicine, it is also a mild and gentle herb for babies; the tea has historically been used for its sedative effects and affinity for the digestive system in treating colic and upset stomachs, dispelling gas, and relieving general stomach ailments and nausea.

The names catnip and catmint are often used interchangeably, yet they are two different plants within the genus *Nepeta* with similar medicinal uses. Catnip can be used to ease stomach and menstrual cramps and promote digestion. In France, the leaves were used for teas before the arrival of tea from China, and it is used in savory and meat dishes alongside more common culinary herbs like thyme and sage. The Cherokee used a poultice of catnip on hives and inflamed skin.

To make a tea for head tension, blend ¼ cup dried lemon balm, ¼ cup dried meadowsweet, 2 tablespoons dried catnip, 2 tablespoons dried chamomile, and 1 tablespoon dried lavender in a jar. For each cup, steep 1 tablespoon of the herb mix in 8 fluid ounces of boiling water for 10 minutes. Drink three times a day for continuing headaches.

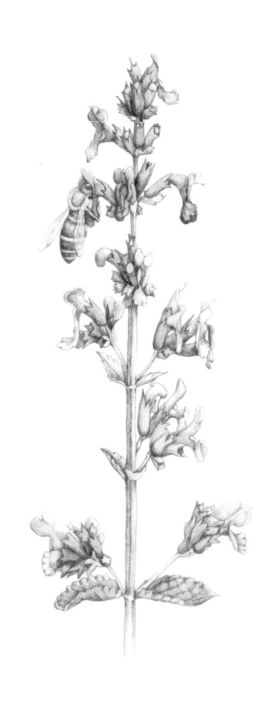

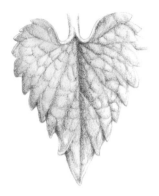

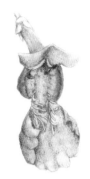

Plant family
Lamiaceae

Other names
Catmint

Region
Native to temperate regions throughout Africa, Asia, and Europe; introduced to North America by European settlers and now widespread in gardens

---

Botanical description
A perennial flowering mint, the roots send up 2- to 3-foot-high plants. Square stems, commonly found in the Lamiaceae family with branched stems. Heart-shaped, toothed leaves have a soft, downy texture. The flowers grow in white whorls sometime dotted with purplish-red spots that terminate at the end of the stem and bloom July to late September.

Grow
Easily grown perennial, catnip often can take over a garden bed, much like other mints, and thus would do well in a pot. Use in borders to deter rodents in the garden and as a trap plant for cats and insects alike.

Gather
Flowering tops in July and August

Herbal actions
Carminative, sedative, diaphoretic, antispasmodic, emmenagogue, tonic, nervine

---

Energetics
Pungent, warming and cooling

Flower essence
Calming for those who feel socially anxious, increases bonds of friendship, and helps in times of transition

---

Preparations
Herbal teas, eaten fresh in salads, infused vinegars or honeys

Chamomile MATRICARIA CHAMOMILLA

*C*hamomile is a herbaceous plant that has naturalized in one of our garden beds, where I often plant the brassicas. Chamomile acts as a companion plant; it deters pests and attracts beneficial insects. Chamomile self-seeds, and its little green fronds pop up shortly after the snow melts. I like to sit and pick the heads of sunny chamomile, raking my fingers gently through the plant. You can also employ a flower rake for large patches.

Chamomile's bitter nature cannot be ascertained from its sweet smell. Used in everything from cosmetics to aromatherapy to beverages, this is the perfect plant for smoothing life's rough edges. Chamomile is a nervine and helps you digest, process, and calm both the mind and the digestive system, the seat of the solar plexus chakra. The solar plexus is connected to your identity, self-esteem, confidence, and self-worth. Chamomile holds whatever comes up for you in a safe space, helping you digest it. Chamomile is particularly good for bloating and nervous feelings in the gut and for cooling overheated systems.

Chamomile holds a sweet, radiant energy and helps us soothe our inner child to process those wounds that are hard to touch. Chamomile is supportive of the skin, reducing inflammation and promoting regeneration of damaged skin. In a spiritual sense, chamomile protects the spirit, perhaps that is why it also allows the body to rest a little easier.

Chamomile is a gentle yet fierce ally for children and is wonderful as a tea. It can be given to young children to soothe anxiety and calm them in times of illness, sleeplessness, aches, and pains from colds and flus and the cramping associated with upset stomachs. It pairs well with lemon balm. I love to rub chamomile infused in oil on little ones' feet to calm them before bed. Externally it can be used as a wash and in herbal baths, as well as for insect bites and sunburns.

CAUTION: Contraindicated if you have allergies to other members of the Asteraceae family (like ragweed).

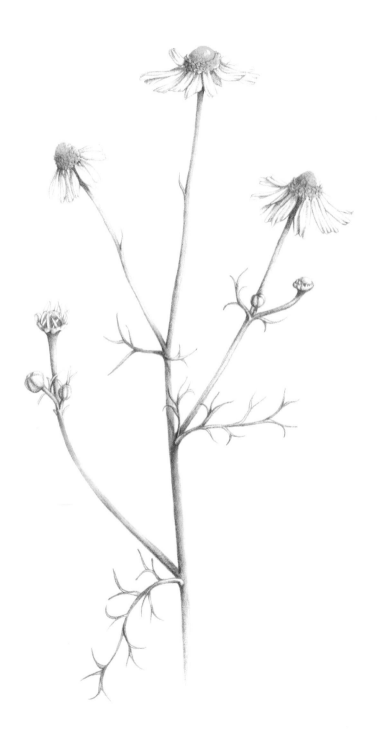

Plant family
Asteraceae

Other names
Mayweed, German chamomile, wild chamomile, ground apple, mother's daisy, Babuna

---

Region
Native to southwestern Asia, southern and eastern Europe; cultivated in India for 200 years; today it is found all over the world.

Botanical description
White ray flowers about ¾ inch wide or inflorescences and yellow disk floret in a compact head that reaches for the sun; pleasant and calming fragrance with bitter taste; ferny, airy green leaves with their own refreshing aroma; low-growing plant

---

Herbal actions
Anti-inflammatory, antimicrobial, antispasmodic, bitter, carminative, nervine

---

Energetics
Bitter, cooling, and drying

Flower essence
For those easily upset or irritable, brings emotional balance

---

Gather
The flowers should be harvested between May and August, while they are dry.

Grow
USDA Hardiness Zones 3–9. Minute seeds grow either in well-balanced or poor soils; direct-seed in the spring or autumn for blooms in the following summer. In my garden, it is a self-seeding perennial. To transplant, start seeds indoors four to six weeks before the last frost. Chamomile needs light to germinate; scatter seeds on top of soil or press in gently—do not cover with soil; it should germinate within 7 to 14 days. When chamomile plant has grown 2 to 3 inches tall, plant outside after the last frost.

Preparations
Infused oils, tisanes, teas, essential oils

Chickweed STELLARIA MEDIA

*F*ound in cool conditions and disturbed soils and on the woods' edge or in a garden bed, in shade and sun, it has been said there is no part of the world where chickweed is not found. It can be foraged in wild and urban areas as well as in your garden beds. Folklore says when chickweed's leaves fold up, rain is on its way.

Likewise, chickweed is a medicinal as well as a mild-tasting nutritive edible, restorative to many systems in the body. It is nutrient dense and high in vitamins A, B, and C, magnesium, manganese, zinc, and potassium—more so than spinach or kale. It helps eliminate waste in the body, detoxifies the blood, and soothes inflammation.

Chickweed is a soothing and moving plant. As the moon moves the tides, chickweed moves emotions and fluids in our bodies. Like the night sky, its flowers resemble our stars and constellations. Chickweed helps you release negative feelings and it releases stagnant lymph. It soothes the soul as well as inflamed tissues, whether in the throat or skin. This plant should not be used for damp skin conditions, but it is potent topical medicine for hot skin conditions such as burns, rashes, eczema, hives, and stings and a wonderful food for hot summer days, such as in a pesto or a summer smoothie.

I often find chickweed again in autumn growing at our woods' edge; it lies in wait under the snow. Chickweed will return when temperatures reach the forties consistently, and it is prone to wilt in hot summer temperatures. Chickweed soothes our emotional states and long-held anger, detoxifying the heat and bringing openness to the heart for forgiveness.

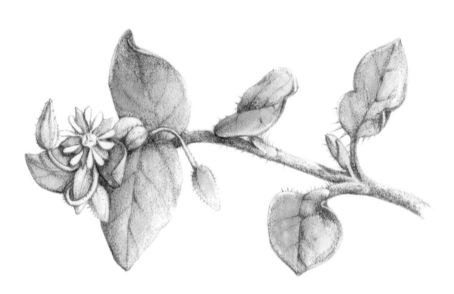

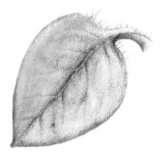

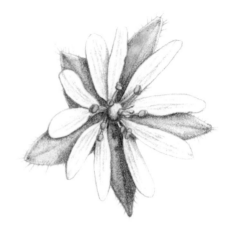

Plant family
Caryophyllaceae

Herbal actions
Tonic, demulcent, alterative, anti-inflammatory, laxative, diuretic, analgesic

Energetics
Cooling

Gather
Cut bunches with scissors from uncontaminated soils throughout spring, summer, and fall. Best eaten right after harvesting or dry for later use.

Flower essence
A plant of the moon, chickweed helps us release negative feelings and soothe angsty emotional states.

Region
Grows throughout the world; brought from Europe, it is widely found across much of North America.

Grow
USDA Hardiness Zones 2–11; it grows well in a variety of climates in containers or right in the garden; prefers moist soils. Plant seeds outdoors directly into the ground in late spring or grow in pots on a sunny windowsill year-round.

Botanical description
Sticks close to the ground, with small, ovate, and smooth opposite leaves; leaves around the base of the flower have fine hairs. Flowers are quite tiny, with five white petals with five green sepals. A single line of hairs runs along the stems.

Preparations
Edible and delicious in salads when young; older more fibrous stalks can be blended into pesto, tossed into smoothies, juiced, or used in infused oils, topical poultices, and teas.

Chickweed and Walnut Pesto

I love to serve this nutritive pesto mixed into pasta or risotto, on pizza in lieu of tomato sauce, or on top of a fish or chicken dish.

1 cup chickweed

3 garlic cloves

¼ cup toasted walnuts

1 tablespoon sea salt

Freshly ground black pepper

Juice of 1 lemon

¼ cup olive oil

*Makes
1 cup*

Pulse the chickweed, garlic, and walnuts in a food processor until coarsely chopped. Add the salt, pepper to taste, and lemon juice, and slowly drizzle in olive oil until emulsified and well combined.

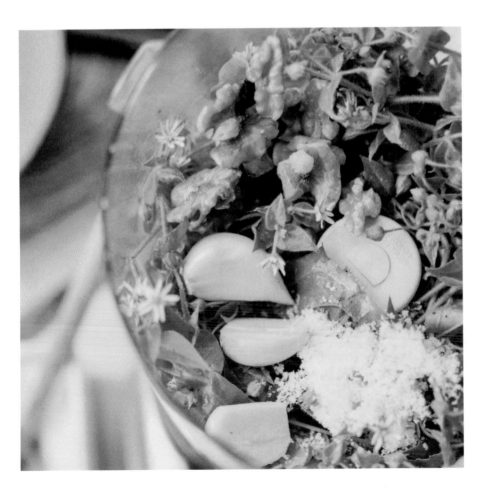

Elder SAMBUCUS NIGRA

*F*or me, elderflowers are pure magic, their blossoms threaded throughout folklore and myth as being portals to other realms. Their arrival is a portal for me, signaling the height of midsummer, blooming along roadsides in a hedgerow, in gardens, at woodland's edge. There is nothing like their fragrant blooms on a warm summer evening breeze. I take caution when plucking clusters so as not to break branches.

Elderflowers are cooling, unbelievably fragrant, sweet little blooms. Ideally taken at the onset of a cold or flu, elderflowers are diaphoretic, clearing heat and promoting sweating, with an affinity for the upper respiratory tract. It is perfect for cooling down your system on increasingly hot summer days. As well as crafting with fresh elderflowers, I dry and save elderflowers for teas to help bring down winter fevers. Elderflowers treat heat-induced respiratory complaints such as coughing, wheezing, sinus congestion, and nasal discharge as well as fevers associated with a cold.

Elderflowers can be used to relieve oppressive and heavy emotional states, especially when one is experiencing stagnation; think moving emotional states like moving a fever out of the body. Elderflower is said to calm anxiety and fears, bringing joy, protection, and prosperity, imbuing one with optimism and resilience.

CAUTION: There are many flowering plants with creamy white blooms, including cowbane and cow parsley, as well as other toxic members of the carrot family (Apiaceae) that have tiny white flowers. The key to identifying the latter is that they grow from the ground, unlike elder, a treelike shrub. If elder is taken in addition to diabetes medication, monitor blood sugar, as there is some concern that elderflower can lower blood sugar.

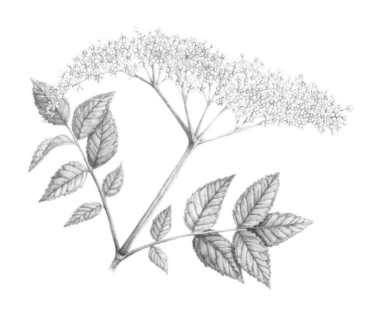

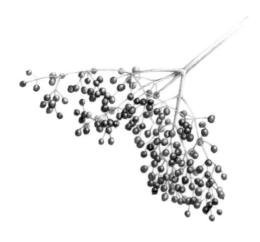

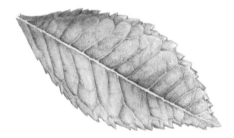

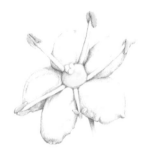

Plant family
Adoxaceae

Region
Grows throughout the world. Native to the Northern Hemisphere.

Botanical description
Elderflowers grow from a woody bush with light gray branches, not the ground, which is one way to distinguish them from some of their toxic look-alikes. Ovate, serrated leaves commonly found in groupings of five to seven. Before elder blooms, it has tight buds that grow larger before creamy-colored sprays of flowers on an umbel with a pale green stalk open. The flowers have five stamens, five petals, and a distinctive floral aroma.

Herbal actions
Diuretic, anti-inflammatory, antispasmodic, nervine, alterative, diaphoretic

Energetics
Cooling and drying

Flower essence
Renewal from the light within; reconnecting with innocence and joy within

Parts used
Flowers and berries

Gather
In May, June, and July when the buds are freshly opened. I leave a fair number of elderflowers on the bush so I can return to harvest elderberries at the end of summer and beginning of fall. Stick with creamy white-colored blooms; if they are starting to turn brown, they are past their prime.

Preparations
Dried for tea, cordials, flavorings, and cakes

Elderflower Cream in a Strawberry Tart

Elderflowers bring me into the moment. Plucking tiny, twinkling white flowers one by one puts me into a midsummer trance and reminds me to savor the moment, because it is so fleeting. What other things are fleeting in our lives? Memories and experiences that we felt would last forever. This recipe is a nod to my study-abroad experience in Paris, where I could walk out my door and find myself in a patisserie. I enjoyed every moment and every bite of that magical experience of self-exploration, which I was so grateful to have. Elderflower cream makes a strawberry tart out of this world.

1 cup whole milk

1 vanilla bean,
halved lengthwise

10 fresh elderflower heads

3 large egg yolks

¼ cup plus 1 tablespoon
granulated sugar or honey
(I prefer honey)

2 tablespoons plus 1¼ cups
all-purpose flour

2 ounces (4 tablespoons)
cold unsalted butter,
cut into pieces

Ice water

1 pint fresh, ripe strawberries,
hulled and sliced

Makes 8 to 10 servings

In a small, heavy-bottomed saucepan, scald the milk with the vanilla bean and elderflowers over medium-high heat. Remove from the heat, cover the pan with a lid, and let the mixture infuse for 15 to 20 minutes.

In a bowl, whisk together 2 of the egg yolks with ¼ cup of the sugar and whisk in 2 tablespoons of the flour.

Strain the vanilla bean and elderflowers from the milk through a mesh strainer and discard the solids. Slowly whisk the infused milk ¼ cup at a time into the yolk mixture to temper. Return the milk mixture to the pan and bring to a boil over medium heat, whisking continuously. Lower heat and continue to cook, whisking for a minute or two more, until the mixture has thickened.

Pour the elderflower cream into a bowl, pressing plastic wrap onto the surface to prevent a skin from forming, and let cool. Then refrigerate until ready to assemble.

Preheat the oven to 400°F.

In a food processor fitted with a blade, process the remaining 1¼ cups flour, the butter, and the remaining 1 tablespoon sugar until the dough forms little balls. Add the remaining egg yolk and, with processor running, add 2 to 3 tablespoons of ice water, just until the dough begins to hold together. Form into a ball and flatten into a disk about ¼ inch thick. Refrigerate for 30 minutes.

Place the dough between two sheets of wax paper and roll it out to a thickness of ⅛ inch.

Line a 9-inch tart mold with a removable bottom with the pastry dough. Prick the dough with a fork and line it with parchment paper and pie weights (I use dried beans). Bake for 12 to 15 minutes, or until golden brown.

Allow the crust to cool completely. To assemble the tart, spread the chilled pastry cream inside the crust and top with the sliced fresh strawberries.

Refrigerate overnight or enjoy immediately!

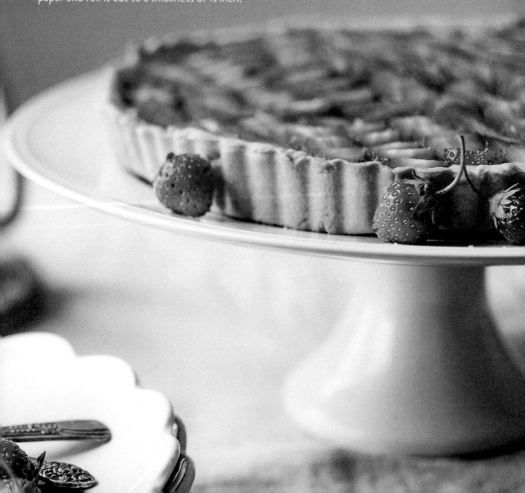

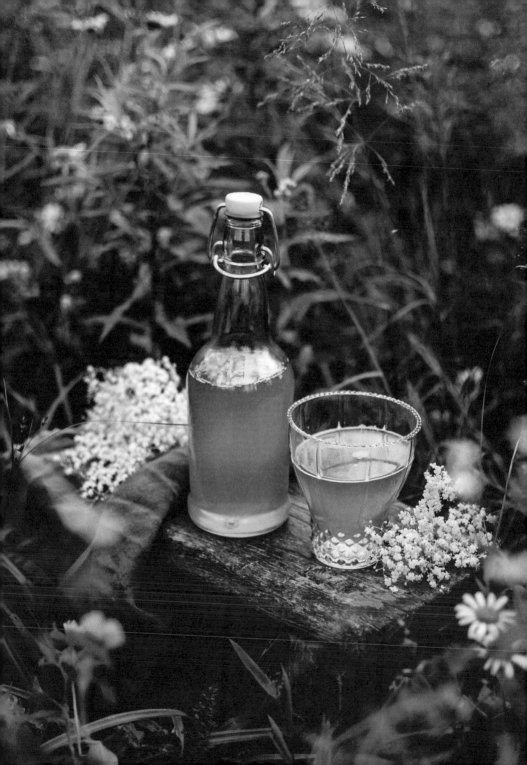

Elderflower Cordial

Pick elderflowers from the bushes and set aside outside to allow any insects to escape before using them. Work with the elderflowers closely after harvesting to retain the fragrance.

20 to 30 heads of elderflowers

1 liter filtered water

4 cups granulated sugar

3 organic lemons

Zest of 1 lemon

2 teaspoons citric acid

Makes 2 bottles

Remove the little white flowers from the green stalks, placing the blossoms in a larger bowl. Remove as much of the stems as possible. In a medium saucepan, boil water, add sugar and stir until it is dissolved, then simmer for 5 more minutes.

Juice the lemons, straining the liquid. Add the juice of the lemons and the citric acid to the pan, and bring to a simmer over medium heat. Remove from heat and let cool. Pour this liquid over your elderflowers, add lemon zest, cover with a tea towel, and let sit at room temperature for 8 to 24 hours.

Sterilize glass bottles and warm them with hot water.

Using a funnel, pour cordial into the sterilized bottles or glass jars and allow to cool. Store for up to 6 months. You can water-bath the bottle to seal for a longer shelf life. Once the bottle is open, refrigerate it and use within 3 weeks. I use 3 tablespoons of cordial in bubbly water or champagne and to sweeten desserts.

Elderflower and Champagne Currant Shrub

This is my favorite shrub or herbal drinking vinegar. I always lament that I don't it make more often the week in summer both elderflowers and currants are ripe, but I save currants for currant jam as well. If you don't have currants growing in your garden, you can check for them at your local farmers' market. If I don't see them, I always ask the farmers at the different stands for a good lead. There are many ways to make a shrub or drinking vinegar. I learned this method from my friend Rachel, I find it convenient and delicious.

1 cup elderflowers, stems removed

1 cup champagne currants

1 cup white wine vinegar or apple cider vinegar

1 cup honey

Sparkling water to serve

Makes 1 quart jar

Muddle the elderflowers and currants in a quart jar and add the vinegar and honey. Mix well with a wooden spoon. Top with a plastic lid or a piece of parchment paper secured with a canning lid. Infuse in the refrigerator for a week, shaking occasionally, then taste. If you'd like a stronger flavor, you can leave it for 2 weeks. Strain the mixture through a sieve lined with cheesecloth and refrigerate. Enjoy 2 tablespoons of shrub over 8 ounces sparkling water and ice.

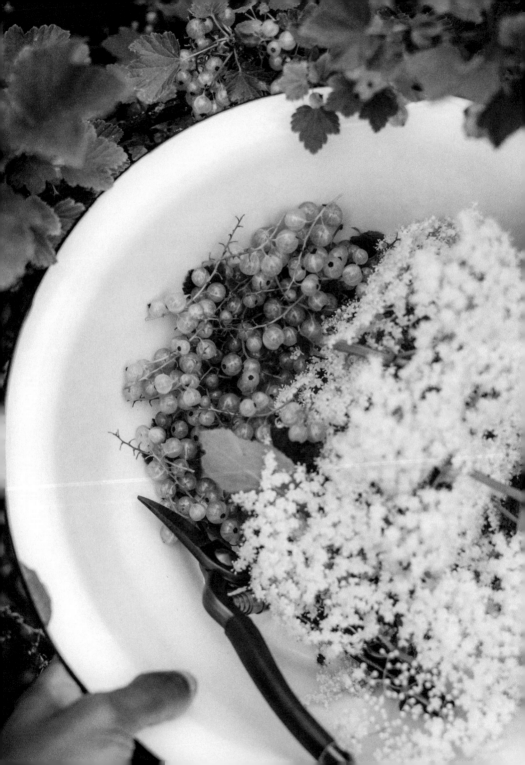

Lavender LAVANDULA ANGUSTIFOLIA

*L*avender puts a pause on racing thoughts and allows the body to rest. Lavender, from the Latin root word *lavare* meaning to wash, washes away tensions and worries, smoothes the muscles of the digestive tract to support the gut-brain axis, lulling one into a more relaxed parasympathetic nervous system state. As a nervine, it can relieve insomnia, depression, anxiety, and headaches. A lavender bath calms the nervous system, soothing one to sleep. An herb for dreamwork, its flowers contain high levels of volatile oils, which are extracted through distillation to create the ever-popular essential oils.

Lavender tea has a similar calming effect as lavender essential oil, which has grown in popularity, but the safety and sustainability of essential oils is still under some debate. It takes so much plant matter to produce one small bottle of essential oils; I'd rather use whole plant material when I can. I sleep nightly with a lavender eye pillow as it calms too much activity and stimulation in the mind, soothing overactivity in the third eye and crown chakra.

Lavender is also used on wounds for its antiseptic properties and can be made into a wound wash. Applied topically, it can also be used to repel insects. Lavender soothes indigestion and relieves gas and bloating.

CAUTION: Lavender is generally safe for both young and old to use. Consuming high amounts may cause headaches, and essential oils should not be applied undiluted on skin.

To make a lavender oil for relaxation, fill a pint-size jar three-quarters of the way with chopped lavender. Add 1½ teaspoons of organic vodka to the chopped lavender and mix, then cover completely with olive oil. Make sure to get all the bubbles out with a chopstick, stir, and cover with the lid. Shake it often. Label the jar with the date and shake it every couple of days. Decant for one moon cycle—4 weeks—and strain the oil through muslin cloth before using.

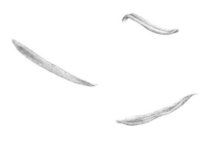

Plant family
Lamiaceae

Region
Native to the Mediterranean area but grows in temperate climates

---

Botanical description
Lavender can grow to be a 2- to 3-foot-tall perennial shrub. It features sage-green opposite leaves with whorls of 6 to 10 violet to blue flowers terminating at the end of a spike.

Grow
Start indoors 8 to 12 weeks before last frost and outdoors 1 to 2 weeks before last frost. This perennial prefers moderately fertile yet well-drained soil and full sun. Here in USDA Hardiness Zone 4B, I grow a cold-hardy variety called Munstead. In the fall, I cover it with a blanket of fallen leaves to protect it from harsh winter winds. In the winter, a blanket of snow is a friend and acts as insulation to help it overwinter.

Gather
Harvest flowering tops when they are in bud stage and hang them in bunches or dry them on screens. From summer into fall, use leaves for herbal infused vinegars.

Herbal actions
Antiseptic, antispasmodic, antidepressant, neuroprotective, antimicrobial, anti-inflammatory, analgesic, nervine, antifungal

---

Energetics
Cooling, drying, bitter

Flower essence
Spiritual sensitivity: Tempers frantic and nervous energy in the nervous system, calms overstimulation in the mind so the physical body can relax.

Preparations
Lavender-infused oils, teas, infusions, lavender latte, essential oil

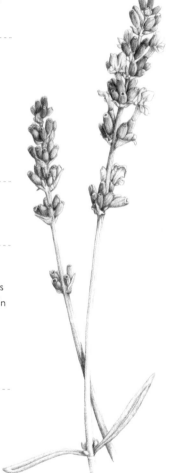

Lavender Honey

This lavender-infused honey can be used to sweeten summer herbal teas and dessert.

¼ cup dried lavender buds, pesticide-free and for culinary use

1 cup honey

Makes 1 cup

Put the lavender buds in a clean, glass pint jar, pour the honey on top, and stir. Make sure the honey and blossoms are well combined. Cover the jar with a lid and place it in a warm spot for one lunar cycle, turning the jar every day and infusing it with your healing intentions and blessings. Once it's ready, strain it through a mesh strainer into a sterilized glass jar and wait a few hours for all the honey to separate. Store in a dark place until ready to use.

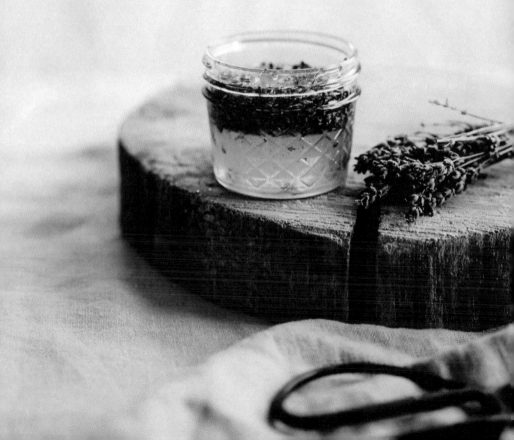

Lavender Pots de Crème

Makes 4 servings

Preheat the oven to 300°F.

Combine the cream and milk in a saucepan over medium heat, bring to a simmer, and remove from the heat. Add the dried lavender, cover the saucepan, and allow the mixture to infuse for 10 minutes. Strain lavender infused milk into a large bowl, add honey and lemon zest. Separate egg yolks. Slowly add a stream of the infused cream into the egg yolks and whisk lightly until smooth and combined. Make sure to avoid cooking the yolks. Add the salt.

Place four small ramekins in a baking dish and pour the mixture, dividing it evenly among the ramekins. Bring water to a boil and carefully pour it around the ramekins (don't splash water into the ramekins) until it reaches up about an inch on the sides of the ramekins. Bake for 40 to 50 minutes until the centers appear firm. Remove from the oven when the middle appears solid and allow to cool completely before serving. Can be prepared ahead of time and refrigerated.

1½ cups heavy cream

½ cup whole milk

2 tablespoons culinary dried lavender or harvested from your garden

⅓ cup honey

1 teaspoon lemon zest

6 large egg yolks

¼ teaspoon kosher salt

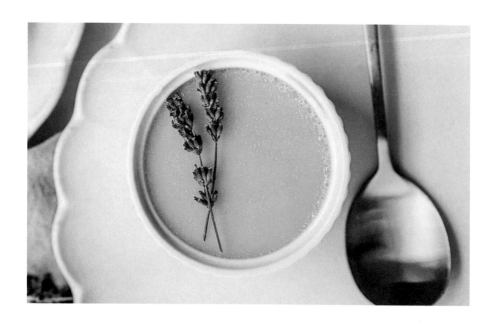

Lemon Balm MELISSA OFFICINALIS

*L*emon balm grows as a perennial in our gardens. Quite like its name, when rubbed between the fingers, it has a lemony aroma. Lemon balm is an herb of joy, vitality, and hope. Working on the nervous system, it helps us connect to the sweetness of life, allowing our bodies to find parasympathetic rest. Lemon balm helps us relax and digest.

Lemon balm is good for tension and anxiety in the body, particularly in the solar plexus and the enteric nervous system; it acts to help tone the vagus nerve and imparts a sense of safety. Uplifting the spirits in seasonal affective disorder and depression, it can be used in conjunction with medications for anxiety connected to the stomach. It spreads voraciously in a garden and is a source of stored sunlight on somber winter days. I collect the leaves all season long to dry for tea and infusions. Lemon balm can be planted as an ornamental or in a pot. It is wonderful for attracting bees to the garden.

Lemon balm was the first plant I worked with in an intentional way, and it happens to be a plant used in Haitian culture, known as melis in Haitain Kreyòl. During our first summer in our cottage, I mowed over a patch that had spread into our lawn unbeknownst to me. Immediately I was drawn in by the fragrant citrusy aroma blowing up from under the mower. I identified the plant and decided to make a tincture. I chopped the herb, stuffed it in a jar, poured vodka over, labeled it, and let it sit on our pantry shelf. Months passed, and I was cleaning out our pantry in the dead of winter when I found the bottles I had made. I gave one to my husband and a friend to try. I tried some drops in my water and instantly felt a sense of ease wash over my body, like sunlight on winter days.

Lemon balm is best used as a tea for purifying the spirits and calming anxiety.

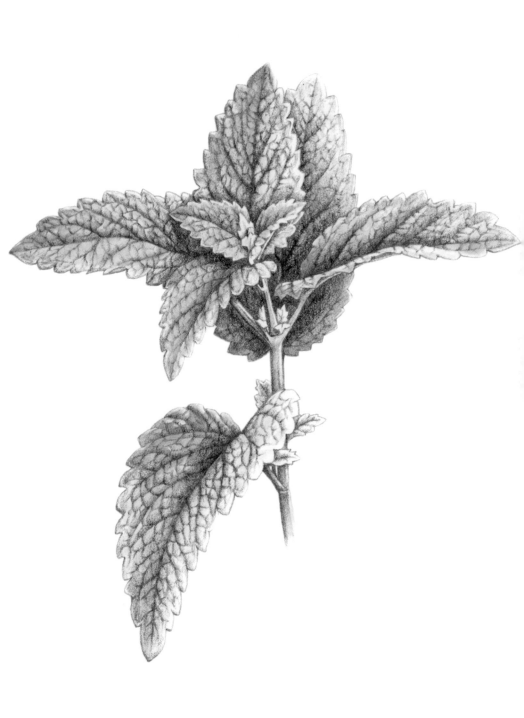

Plant family
Lamiaceae

Other names
Sweet balm, balm mint,
bee herb

Herbal actions
Antiviral, antispasmodic,
antibacterial, diuretic,
nervine, tonic, calming

Energetics
Sweet, cool

Gather
Aerial parts when flowers
open; hang in bunches or
screen dry. Garble, removing
damaged leaves after drying

Region
Native to North Africa, the
Mediterranean, Iran, and
central Asia, it is cultivated all
over the world.

Flower essence
Brings in balance and
relaxation when we're
stretched thin; lets go of grief
to have a joyful heart

Grow
USDA Hardiness Zones 4–9.
Easily grown from seed. start
indoors 6 to 8 weeks before
the last frost or outdoors 2 to
3 weeks before. This mint
family perennial herb prefers
rich and well-drained soil and
grows well in sun with some
afternoon shade. Drought
tolerant once established. It
grows well in a container,
especially to keep it from
spreading.

Botanical description
Soft, green heart-shaped
leaves with scalloped edges.
When in bloom, it features
small white flowers on the
square stems.

Preparations
Infusions, tinctures, culinary
use, teas, honey, simple
syrups, ice cream, pesto,
powdered, infused in oil

Roasted Lemon Balm Chicken with Herbed Butter

I love a well-seasoned roasted chicken to use in salads. I use the bones for nourishing broth (page 299). This recipe employs summer's abundant and citrusy herb, lemon balm, to impart a novel and herbal twist.

Makes 5 to 7 servings

Preheat the oven to 400°F. Divide the lemon balm, thyme sprigs, and sage leaves in half and set one half aside. Chop the remaining herbs and mix them thoroughly in a bowl with the butter.

Loosen the skin of the chicken and rub butter mixture under the skin of chicken and place it in a roasting pan. Season the skin with salt and pepper and rub olive oil on top. Place the reserved herbs and 1 of the garlic halves in the cavity of the chicken. Tie the legs together with kitchen string.

Scatter the lemon quarters and the remaining 3 garlic halves around the chicken and pour the wine in the pan. Roast for 45 minutes, until golden brown and internal temperature reads 165°F on a meat thermometer. Remove from the oven, scatter the chopped carrots in the pan, and continue to roast for another 30 minutes, until juices run clear.

½ cup fresh lemon balm leaves

6 fresh thyme sprigs

¼ cup fresh sage leaves

¼ cup salted butter, at room temperature

1 whole chicken

Salt and freshly ground black pepper

Extra virgin olive oil

2 garlic cloves, halved crosswise or smashed

2 lemons, quartered

½ to 1 cup white wine or chicken broth

4 carrots, chopped

Raspberry and Lemon Balm Compote

Makes 1 pint jar

In small mixing bowl, combine the lemon balm and boiling water. Steep for 10 minutes. Cool, strain the lemon balm leaves, and add the raspberries, honey, orange juice, and let sit for 5 minutes. Pour the mixture into a medium saucepan and bring to a boil, then lower the heat to medium-low and simmer until the mixture has thickened, about ten minutes. Ladle into a clean pint jar, cover, and store in refrigerator for up to 2 weeks. Serve atop a bowl of porridge or toast or vanilla ice cream.

2 tablespoons lemon balm leaves

½ cup boiling water

2 cups raspberries, fresh or frozen

¼ cup honey

1 tablespoon orange juice

VARIATION: Substitute blueberries for raspberries and lavender for lemon balm.

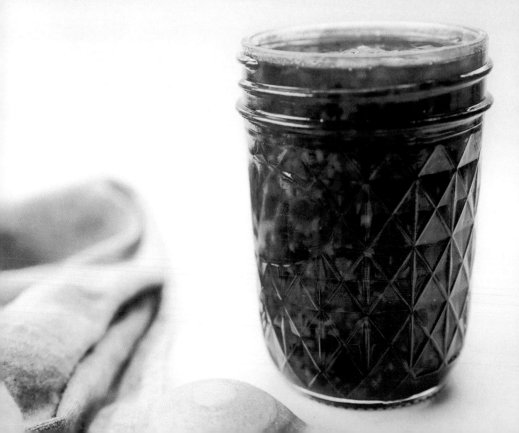

Linden TILIA SPP.

*L*inden is a gentle balm for frayed nerves in hot summer heat, a plant for urban and suburban foragers alike. Used simply in a hot infusion, it was employed in Europe and by the Potawatomi, Cherokee, and Iroquois Native American tribes in a variety of uses, including for gastrointestinal problems and calming anxiety of the mind. It can be used in a soothing bath or soak to bring down restlessness and nerves. In traditional Chinese medicine, linden is said to calm the shen, or the energy of the heart. Linden's heart-shaped leaves point to its effects on the physical and emotional heart, and it has a relaxing effect on the circulatory system and hypertension. In folk medicine, linden was used for the flu, coughs, and migraines.

The mucilaginous, or demulcent, effects combined with its nervine properties makes it a balm for nervous tension in the digestive system and for sore throats.

TO MAKE AN INFUSION, steep I to 2 teaspoons of dried flowers in 8 ounces boiling water for 30 minutes. Linden pairs well with lemon balm and hawthorn leaves and flowers.

CAUTION: The flowers may cause allergic reactions to those with allergies to tree species.

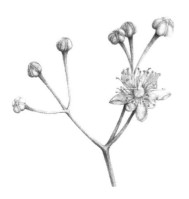
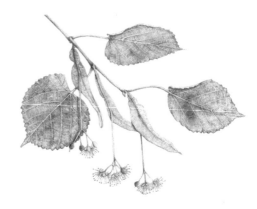

Plant family
Tiliaceae

Other names
Linden, basswood, duan shu hua (TCM), lime flower

Region
Varieties easily grow in northern and temperate climates of Europe, North America, and Asia; many medicinal varieties are known, with *Tilia cordata*, *T. platyphyllos*, and *T. americana* being the most available and well known.

Botanical description
Deciduous tree growing up to 100 feet tall; gray bark; heart-shaped leaves with leaf bract and fragrant flower cluster of white to yellowish flowers

---

Herbal actions
Nervine, diuretic, relaxant, antispasmodic, diaphoretic, demulcent, anxiolytic

---

Energetics
Cooling, drying, moistening

Flower essence
Helps with relaxing into new paths and releasing emotional blocks; opens our hearts to feel connectedness

Gather
Harvest flowers and bracts from trees when they are dry (at least 24 hours after a rainfall) and after a few blossoms in a cluster have opened for peak fragrance (they bloom over a period of 2 weeks). This is best done in the morning before the noon sun dries the flowers.

Preparations
Tinctures, tea, infused honey, bath

Meadowsweet FILIPENDULA ULMARIA

*T*he fragrance of meadowsweet flowers is reminiscent of marzipan carried on the breeze, an olfactory delight. Their taste is even sweeter infused into jams, desserts, and beverages. Meadowsweet's name portends to where it can be found: in meadows, wet soils, damp woods, and at marshes' edges. In our garden, meadowsweet lives under the dappled light of our apple tree, nestled between elder and compass plants. In midsummer, the plumes of micro flowers are abuzz with honeybees.

The essence of meadowsweet reminds us to stay open and receptive to the sweetness of life, how to remain open to channel awareness and to rid ourselves of the idea of separateness. Meadowsweet traditionally was used as a remedy for pain as it contains salicylic acid. In the late 1890s, this compound was isolated in meadowsweet and developed into aspirin. The isolated chemical derived from meadowsweet leaves in an extract, however, was upsetting on the stomach. Combine with chamomile or plantain for a balanced formula to soothe the digestive tract.

Like other members of the Rosaceae (rose) family, you can use meadowsweet for upset stomachs. Its cooling nature helps with hot headaches, moving stagnant energy in the head during summer heat waves. Meadowsweet was among the sacred herbs used by ancient Druids and can be used in a potpourri, retaining its fragrance for many months.

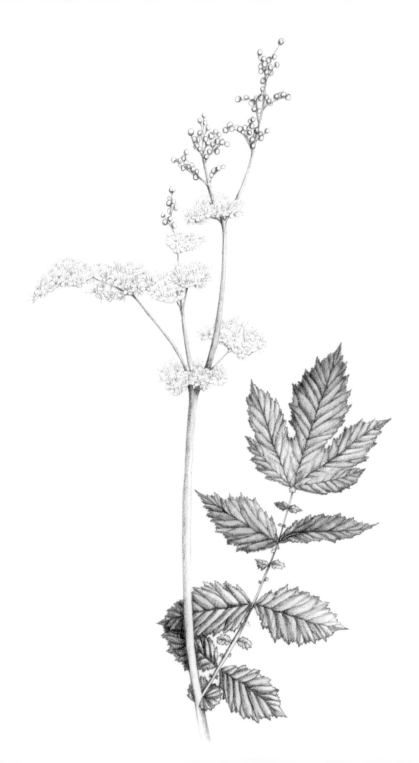

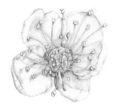

Plant family
Rosaceae

- - - - - - - - - - - - - - - - - - -

Other names
Bridewort, meadwort, lady of the meadow

- - - - - - - - - - - - - - - - - - -

Region
Native to Europe, from Britain to Iceland, and naturalized through temperate Asia, North America, and Australia

- - - - - - - - - - - - - - - - - - -

Botanical description
Creamy, almond-scented flowers with five petals and many sepals atop long, rounded stems. Meadowsweet grows from the ground nearly 3 feet tall. Leaves are made of alternating sets of large and small leaves set opposite each other on the red stem.

- - - - - - - - - - - - - - - - - - -

Herbal actions
Cooling, astringent, analgesic, diaphoretic, anti-inflammatory, tonic

- - - - - - - - - - - - - - - - - - -

Energetics
Cool, bitter, dry

- - - - - - - - - - - - - - - - - - -

Flower essence
Meadowsweet flower essence helps us open to receive and teaches us how to be gentle with ourselves.

Gather
Leaves in the spring, flowers in midsummer to fall

- - - - - - - - - - - - - - - - - - -

Grow
Best sown outdoors in late winter / early spring or can be divided in later autumn or winter.

- - - - - - - - - - - - - - - - - - -

Preparations
Leaves in teas or infusions, flowers in tea and lemonades and to flavor desserts

Meadowsweet Lemonade

Lemonades in summer are refreshing. The addition of cooling herbs and summer florals gives even more potency to this summer brew. Meadowsweet brings relief in the sweltering heat. This method can be used with elderflowers and roses as well.

Makes 4 servings

Mix all the ingredients including the sliced lemon together in a one liter jar. Top with a lid. Infuse 4 to 6 hours, or overnight. Strain and refrigerate. Enjoy the lemonade over ice with a slice of lemon.

5 fresh meadowsweet heads, stems removed

Juice of 1 lemon

⅓ cup honey

4 cups water

1 teaspoon apple cider vinegar

1 lemon, sliced

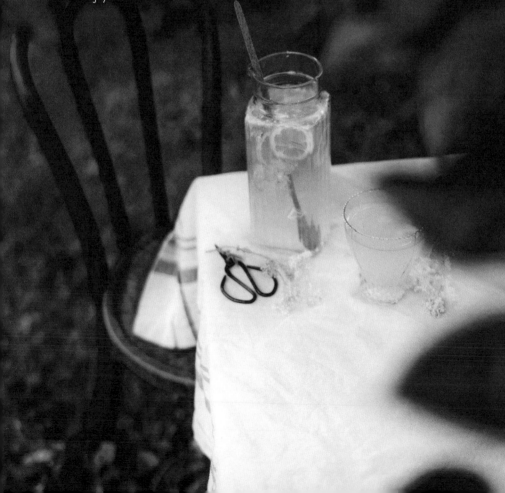

Monarda MONARDA FISTULOSA

B ee balm flowers in late July, dotting our prairie and often covered in buzzing, contented bumblebees. A native plant to the Americas, it was a primary healing plant of many Indigenous tribes. Used by the Wisconsin Ho-Chunk in a sweat bath, its aroma eases cold symptoms via steam inhalation.

Also known as wild oregano or wild bergamot, bee balm is important ecologically to grow and cultivate in North American gardens because it is a native species and a friend to the bees. Monarda's leaves contain thymol, a compound found in thyme and oregano that is antibacterial and stimulating, making it a favorite in our family for winter teas that are comforting for colds and flus. It soothes fevers, headaches, and digestive issues. The blooms and the leaves are spicy and a delicious, pungent addition to pesto and salads. *Monarda didyma* has a milder flavor than the spicy *M. fistulosa*.

As a flower essence, it is used for grounding, energy moving, clearing, connecting to the collective, and helping one clear out old stories and belief systems. It opens the way to plant new intentions and rewrite storylines for the heart and mind.

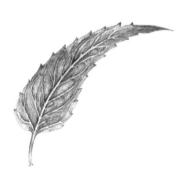

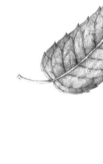

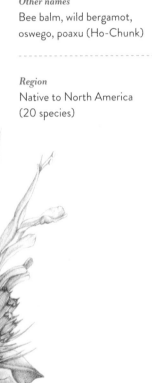

Plant family
Lamiaceae

Other names
Bee balm, wild bergamot,
oswego, poaxu (Ho-Chunk)

Region
Native to North America
(20 species)

Botanical description
Square stem and opposing
leaves, a trademark of the
Lamiaceae family. *Monarda
fistulosa* has purple to white
flowers; *M. didyma* flowers are
a dark red color.

Grow
Perennial, grows in clay soils;
prone to powdery mildew in
late summer

Gather
Harvest the blooms and
leaves in July or August.

Herbal actions
Antiseptic, carminative,
diuretic, antibacterial,
antifungal, antiviral,
antispasmodic, diaphoretic

Energetics
Pungent and warming

Flower essence
Clearing out stagnant beliefs

Preparations
Dried for teas, in salads,
pesto, oxymel, herbal steam

Monarda Oxymel

Derived from a Greek word meaning "acid and honey," an oxymel is an herbal preparation using apple cider vinegar and soothing honey. Both have properties to boost immunity and improve digestion as well as getting the herbal constituents of the plant used.

½ cup dried monarda flowers and leaves

1 cup organic apple cider vinegar

1 cup raw honey (local if you can find it)

Makes 1 pint jar

Fill a pint-size jar one-quarter full with dried monarda. Cover with one part vinegar and one part honey. Stir the mixture and cover it with a plastic lid or a piece of parchment paper under a metal lid. Shake until well mixed and store in a dark place, shaking every couple days. Make this on a new moon and decant on a full moon, or over the course of a 2-week period. Strain the mixture through a mesh strainer lined with cheesecloth, squeezing out as much liquid as possible, and pour the strained oxymel into a glass pint-size jar or bottle. Label it with date and description and store in a cool dark place for up to 6 months. Add a tablespoon or two to warm water during cold and flu season or to salad dressings or to bubbly water on a hot day (remember that a sour taste is cooling).

NOTE
You can experiment with herbs here like garlic, lemon balm, dandelion, nettle, elecampane, mullein, holy basil—the list and experiments are endless.

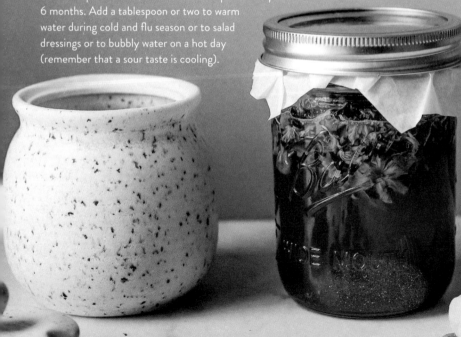

Multiflora Rose

ROSA MULTIFLORA, ROSA RUGOSA

A perennial plant found in gardens, abandoned agricultural land, along roads and the forest's edge, and in prairie thickets, multiflora rose spreads through its running roots. It is categorized throughout North America as a "noxious weed" because it crowds agricultural pastures and irritates cattle. A true wild rose is single flower with five petals, unlike the multi-petaled garden rose. Its hips are a vital winter wildlife food and provides shelter for bears, deer, coyotes, hares and rabbits, chipmunks, and birds.

Multiflora rose, or wild rose, is considered an invasive species, but this is one case when I wonder if a plant has arrived because it is a medicine we need. Multiflora rose is so soothing for the heart space, and it's one of my most favorite remedies for trauma, grief, depression, and heartbreak. Wild rose is a powerful medicine for the heart, especially during times of social upheaval and processing the shadow parts that exist within ourselves and our society. Wild rose nourishes the heart chakra, physically and emotionally.

Wild rose aids in the health of the circulatory system and acts as an aphrodisiac, helping open the body that has a low libido and frigidity. A mood-altering and uplifting plant, bringing cheer and easing heartbreak, wild rose is also edible. It is energetically cooling, used to tone and tighten tissues, easing hot-tissue states like sunburns, swelling, and wounds. Indigenous peoples chewed the leaves as a poultice for bee stings. It is a powerful vulnerary and anti-inflammatory for heat-related skin conditions and wounds (rashes, bites, stings, and abrasions) and also provides pain relief.

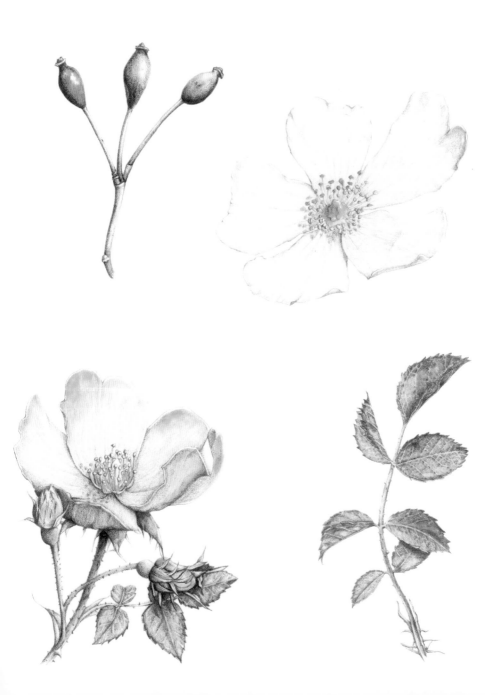

Plant family
Rosaceae

Other names
Prairie rose, dog rose, wild rose, swamp rose, seven sisters rose

---

Varieties
Rosa canina, Rosa rugosa

Region
Native to Japan, Korea, and China, distributed throughout North America and worldwide

Botanical description
Perennial shrub or climbing vine with arching stems bearing thorns. Flowers are 1 inch wide with five petals ranging from pink to white with five green sepals at the base bloom in May. Pinnate leaves are deep green with toothed edges and fringed stipules.

Herbal actions
Anti-inflammatory, antispasmodic, astringent, antiseptic, aphrodisiac, cardiovascular tonic, nervine, vulnerary

Energetics
Cooling and drying

Flower essence
Protection, having an open heart with boundaries, emotional safety

---

Gather
The flowers should be harvested in spring and summer; rose hips in the morning of fall months when the resin is sticky and dry.

Preparations
Wild rose honey, shrubs, syrups; flowers are edible.

Wild Rose Infused Honey

This honey is quite delicious in summer iced teas and in my favorite summer salad dressing along with Dijon mustard, red wine vinegar, and marjoram. Wild rose opens the heart, and when sharing a meal that features this ingredient, you can feel the love across the table increasing with every bite.

1 cup wild roses, flowers, petals, and buds

1 cup local honey

Makes 1 half-pint jar

Fill a small jar with enough roses to fill it to the top, but do not pack them too densely. Fill the jar halfway with honey. Use a chopstick to stir the ingredients, releasing any air bubbles or pockets. If your honey is crystallized, you can gently warm it on the stovetop, being careful not to get it too hot, because that can destroy beneficial enzymes in the honey. Add the remainder of the honey, stirring again to ensure all the blossoms are well coated. Cover and infuse for 1 to 2 weeks. You can enjoy a teaspoon of honey in your tea, either leaving the petals or straining them out, as you prefer.

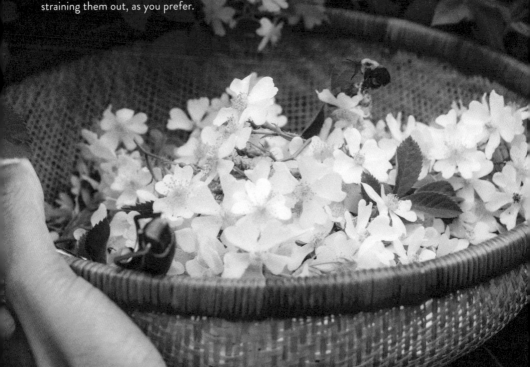

Nasturtium TROPAEOLUM MAJUS

I adore the scallop-circle leaves and cheerful blooms of nasturtiums in my summer garden. I often plant nasturtium betwixt and between the vegetables in my garden for its powerful roles in companion planting and promoting the health of vegetables nearby and for its ability to deter pests. I plant it with my squash and brassicas like cabbage, kale, and broccoli. They do well next to tomatoes, radishes, and cucumbers, too.

Spicy and peppery, nasturtium is a powerful antimicrobial used internally for respiratory infections like bronchitis. As a companion plant, nasturtium serves as a protector in the garden. It repels cucurbit vegetable pests like the squash bug and cucumber beetle and attracts beneficial predatory insects. All parts of this plant are edible: leaves, flowers, and the young seedpods, which can be pickled like a caper. Its warming, peppery flavor and high antioxidants are used for infections in the lungs and the urinary tract. The peppery tasting nasturtium seed was ground up and used as a pepper substitute.

Nasturtiums have broad-spectrum antibacterial, antifungal, antiseptic properties. In folk medicine, it was used for scurvy due to its high vitamin C content and to treat colds, the flu, and muscle pains. In Indigenous South American folkways, particularly Andean herbal medicine, it was used to heal wounds and as an expectorant for chest congestion and clearing phlegm. The leaves and flowers are steeped in hot water for digestive tea and respiratory infections.

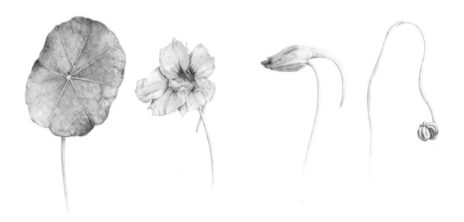

Plant family
Tropaeolaceae

Other names
Peruvian or Mexican cress

Region
Native to South America and Central America; cultivated in gardens worldwide

Botanical description
Climbing annual; rounded leaves and orange, yellow, red, or pink trumpet flowers with a long spur

Grow
In USDA Hardiness Zones 2–11 as an annual. Direct-seed 2 weeks before last frost or sow indoors 4 to 6 weeks before the last frost, first soaking seeds 4 to 6 hours to speed germination. Plant seeds 1 inch deep; nasturtium seeds like warm soil and do well on a heating pad. Cover seeds as they need darkness to germinate. Full sun to midday shade is welcome by this easy-to-grow plant.

Gather
Flowers, leaves, and undeveloped seedpods

Herbal actions
Antibacterial, antifungal, antiseptic, diuretic, emmenagogue, expectorant, stimulant

Energetics
Warming

Flower essence
Grounds the buzzy feeling in your head into the body; aligns the lower chakras with the head and thinking mind; brings warmth to logic.

Preparations
Infused vinegar; infusion of the leaves; flowers and leaves eaten raw, unripe seeds pickled like capers, leaves ground in oil

Nasturtium, Pecan, and Tomato Salad

For the vinaigrette, whisk together olive oil, vinegar, mustard, lemon juice, honey, and salt to taste in a bowl. Set aside.

To prepare the salad, remove any stems from the nasturtium leaves and flowers. Slice the tomatoes in halves or quarters.

Toss the greens, nasturtium leaves, and shallots together in a bowl or serving dish, Arrange the nasturtium flowers on the greens and top with chopped pecans, halved tomatoes, and feta. Drizzle vinaigrette over the salad and sprinkle with salt and pepper. Serve immediately.

Nasturtium Vinaigrette

½ cup olive oil

2 tablespoons Nasturtium-Infused Vinegar (opposite)

¼ teaspoon Dijon mustard

2 tablespoons lemon juice

1 tablespoon honey

Kosher salt and freshly ground pepper

Salad

1 cup nasturtium leaves

½ cup nasturtium flowers (about 16)

1 cup cherry tomatoes

3 cups mixed greens

1 shallot, thinly sliced

¼ cup toasted, chopped pecans

¼ cup crumbled feta cheese

Kosher salt and freshly ground black pepper

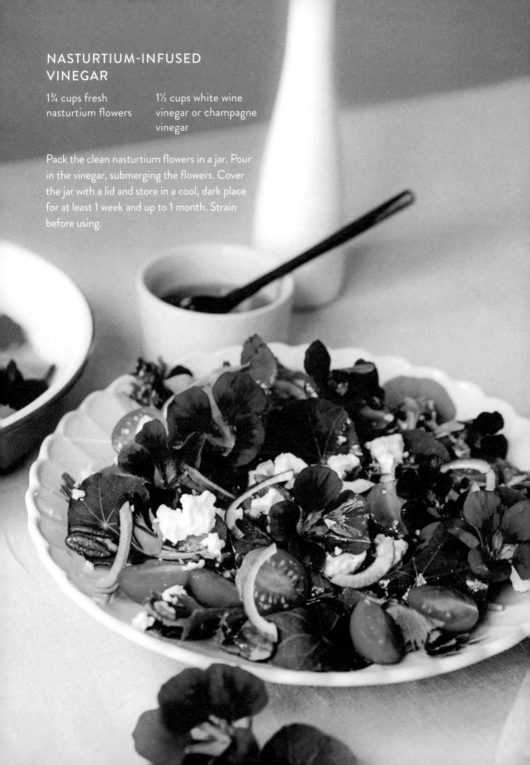

NASTURTIUM-INFUSED VINEGAR

1¾ cups fresh
nasturtium flowers

1½ cups white wine
vinegar or champagne
vinegar

Pack the clean nasturtium flowers in a jar. Pour
in the vinegar, submerging the flowers. Cover
the jar with a lid and store in a cool, dark place
for at least 1 week and up to 1 month. Strain
before using.

Purslane PORTULACA OLERACEA

*B*randed as an unwelcome weed, this unassuming garden plant that grows in driveways, sidewalk cracks, and poor soil is one of the most nutritious plants on this earth. Purslane's consumption as a vegetable dates back at least 2,000 years in Europe and Iran.

Medicinally it is used for urinary and digestive problems because of its mucilaginous, soothing nature. Its high vitamin C content also means immune support. It can be eaten raw and used to thicken soups because of its mucilaginous leaves.

Purslane is an excellent source of omega-3 fatty acids, along with B vitamins, amino acids, calcium, manganese, and phosphorus.

CAUTION: Large amounts can cause an upset stomach, and those with a history of kidney stones should be especially cautious. Do not take medicinally during pregnancy.

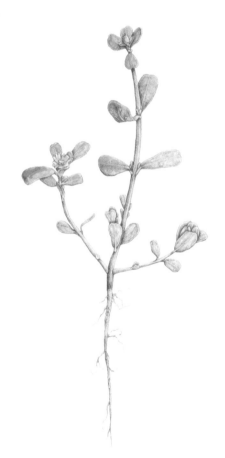

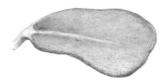

Plant family
Portulacaceae

- -

Other names
Ma chi xian (TCM), verdolaga (Mexico), pourpier (France)

- -

Region
Native to India. Some varieties native to Canada and Greenland; distributed in temperate regions and tropical regions worldwide

Botanical description
Flat, succulent leaves; thick green or red stems; yellow flowers with five petals

- -

Parts used
Leaves and flowers edible

- -

Grow
I've never grown purslane because it seems to appear every spring in my garden.

- -

Gather
Leaves in the morning, from early summer to fall

Herbal actions
Nutritive, anti-inflammatory, antibacterial, diuretic, antioxidant, hypotensive, antiviral

- -

Energetics
Cooling and moistening, sour

- -

Preparations
Eaten raw in salads, cooked in soups as a thickening agent

Purslane and Nettle Dutch Pancake

*Makes 4
servings*

Preheat the oven to 420°F. In a pot of boiling water, add the greens and blanch them for 30 seconds. Drain them immediately, add to a blender, and puree until smooth. In the blender or by hand in a bowl, thoroughly combine the pureed greens, flour, eggs, salt, and pepper. Put the butter in a 10-inch cast-iron pan and place it in the heated oven to melt the butter, then quickly pour the batter into the hot pan, sprinkle the mint and scallions on top, and bake for 20 minutes, or until golden and puffed up.

Meanwhile, make the herbed ricotta in a bowl by mixing all the ingredients together until incorporated.

Remove the pancake from the oven, top with the herbed ricotta, and serve immediately.

¼ cup mixed purslane and nettle leaves

¾ cup all-purpose or gluten-free flour

3 large eggs

½ teaspoon kosher salt

½ teaspoon freshly ground black pepper

3 tablespoons unsalted butter

1 tablespoon chopped fresh mint

1 tablespoon chopped scallions, green parts

Herbed Ricotta

½ cup ricotta cheese

½ teaspoon kosher salt

1 tablespoon chopped scallions, green parts

1 tablespoon chopped thyme

1 tablespoon chopped mint

Rose ROSA DAMASCENA

*T*he garden rose, a symbol of love and object of beauty throughout time. Fossil records show that rose is one of the most ancient flowers, an ancient embodiment of love. Rose supports us in decolonizing our hearts and minds, creating a boundary to soften into our wounds. Rose's love is a boundaried love. The flowers, in shades of red and pink, indicate their use for the blood and the heart that pumps blood throughout our bodies. The supple petals echo softness to our heart space, relieving tensions.

There is a reason we give roses to lovers. The rose is about sharing our love in a container of safety. The nervine actions of roses mean that when we are brokenhearted, rose supports our nervous system, giving us a place to process. Rose relaxes us enough to experience a breath of pleasure and pain. It is a plant for grief and loss, soothing our agitated energies.

Rose is a cooling plant also indicated for fertility, balancing menstruation, and easing congestion in the uterus. A vulnerary, rose's delicious softness and constricting action make it wonderful for the skin and tissue repair and toning, and it has anti-inflammatory properties.

You can make an elderflower and rose facial oil by combining ¼ cup dried rose petals, ¼ cup dried elderflower, and 1 cup sweet almond oil in a clean glass pint jar. Pour 1 cup sweet almond oil over, cover, and infuse for one lunar cycle (4 weeks), shaking every few days. Strain it through a mesh strainer into a clean 8-ounce glass bottle or jar with a tight-fitting lid and store.

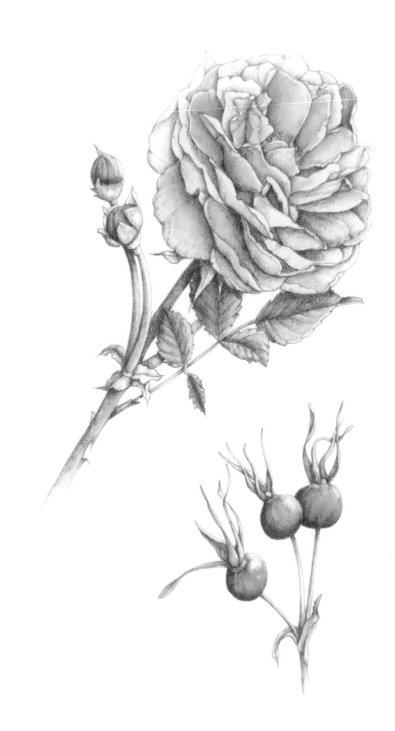

Plant family
Rosaceae

Other name
Garden rose

Region
Native to temperate and subtropic regions in Asia, Europe, and northwest Africa; now cultivated throughout the world

Botanical description
A woody, perennial flowering shrub, climbing or trailing; flowers with 3-inch blooms; smooth petals (often multiple)

Herbal actions
Astringent, nervine, antispasmodic, antimicrobial, anti-inflammatory, antioxidant, vulnerary, reproductive tonic

Energetics
Cooling, drying

Flower essence
Cradling the emotional heart

Gather
Buds and petals are June flowering, I even have a variety that flowers until late fall. Make sure the flowers you are harvesting are not sprayed with pesticides.

Grow
Plant roses in well-drained soil, about 2 feet deep, in a sunny location where they receive six hours of sun per day. They can be propagated from cuttings from an already established rose bush.

Preparations
Infused in honey, baths, jams, teas, hydrosol, creams, tinctures, elixirs

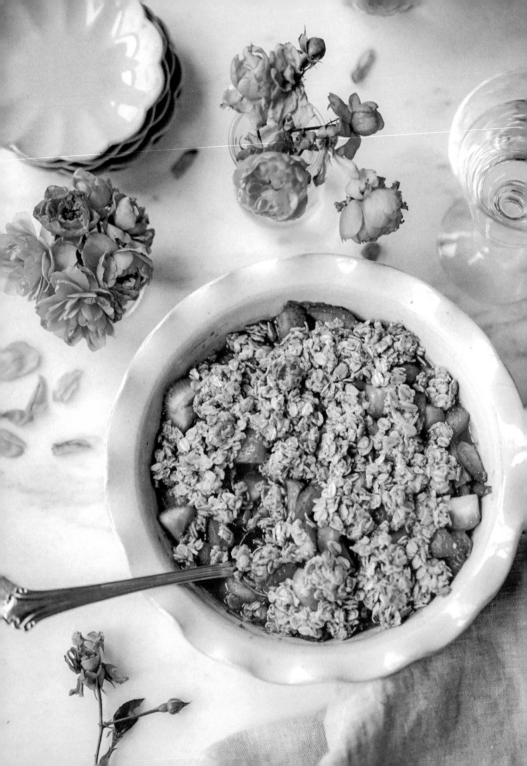

Rhubarb, Rose, and Strawberry Crumble

Rose petals, strawberries, and rhubarb are a seasonal combination that I regularly use in our late-spring/early-summer kitchen. From shrubs to jams to this crumble, the tartness of rhubarb and the sweetness of strawberry and rose pair well together.

Makes 6 to 8 servings

Preheat oven to 375°F and grease a pie dish or 8-inch square dish.

To prepare the filling, in a bowl, combine the rhubarb, strawberries, cornstarch, vanilla extract, rose petals, and rose petal honey in a bowl, stirring gently until well coated, and spoon it into the prepared pie dish in an even layer.

For the topping, in a clean bowl, blend together the rolled oats, almond flour, cinnamon, cardamom, and salt. With a fork or pastry cutter, mix in butter and honey until butter is the size of peas. Sprinkle the topping evenly over the rhubarb filling and bake until the filling is bubbling, and the top is golden brown, 40 to 45 minutes. Let cool for 15 minutes before serving. Top with whipped cream or vanilla bean ice cream.

Filling

3 cups chopped rhubarb

2 cups hulled and sliced strawberries

2 tablespoons cornstarch, flour, or arrowroot powder

1 teaspoon vanilla extract

2 tablespoons rose petals, chopped

¼ cup rose petal honey (powdered rose petals or fresh petals infused in honey)

Topping

1½ cups rolled oats

1¼ cups almond flour (or flour of your choice)

1 teaspoon ground cinnamon

½ teaspoon ground cardamom

¼ teaspoon kosher salt

¼ cup (4 tablespoons) unsalted butter, cold and cubed

¼ to ½ cup honey

Whipped cream or vanilla ice cream, for serving

St. John's Wort

HYPERICUM PERFORATUM

St. John's wort is a woody, weed-like perennial that grows in our front yard garden beds. If you didn't know the treasure you had, you might pull it as a weed. St. John's wort holds the power of the sun at its peak, when the flowers open on the summer solstice, dispelling any darkness of the soul, empowering and supporting our personal will, the sun within, our solar plexus. Found in fields with dry soils, St. John's wort is a well-researched herb used for depression and nerve pain, regenerating the nerve endings and the spirit. The red oil released when the flower is squeezed is an example of the doctrine of signature for healing wounds.

St. John's wort is neuroprotective, helping to improve our ability to reach a parasympathetic state of rest and restore, easing our pain so we can regenerate and sleep better. I love using St. John's wort oil in the winter, rubbing it on the knots in my neck that feel deadened or hardened. I also incorporate St. John's wort into our herbal repertoire for burns, wounds, bruises, and other skin ailments, including the oil in my salves.

CAUTION: St. John's wort can cause photosensitivity if taken internally. Avoid combining it with selective serotonin reuptake inhibitors (SSRIs) and with pharmaceutical drugs, such as birth control, as St. John's wort may reduce the effectiveness of many of these medications. Seek advice from a health-care professional to avoid potential interactions.

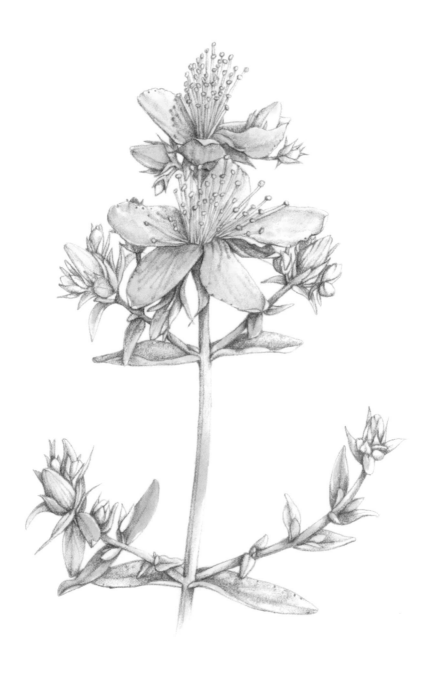

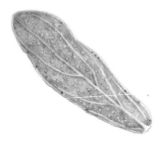

Plant family
Hypericaceae

Other names
Guan ye lian qiao (TCM),
rosin rose, goatweed

Herbal actions
Analgesic, nervine,
antimicrobial, antidepressant,
antiviral, vulnerary, anti-
inflammatory

Energetics
Warming, drying

Gather
Gather unopened buds,
flowering tops, and leaves
from the summer solstice
through fall. Squeeze a bud to
test for the red pigment.

Flower essence
Growing awareness, protects
body from too much light,
anchors consciousness

Region
Naturalized, thriving
worldwide in temperate
regions from Africa, South
America, and Australia; native
to Europe, Asia, North
Africa, and the Middle East;
prefers sunny, well-drained
soils; can be grown from seed

Grow
In USDA Hardiness Zones
3–8. Press seeds on the
surface of the soil indoors
6 to 8 weeks before the last
frost date and transplant after
the last frost has passed and
your seedlings are about
2 inches high, or sow outside
after the danger of frost has

passed; they need light to
germinate. It can grow in
either a container or the
garden and adapts to most
soil conditions.

Botanical description
Yellow star flowers with five
sepals and five petals at the
ends of branching stems;
oblong, opposite leaves that
are perforated with tiny dots
or perforations you can see
when leaves are held up to
the light. When squished, the
buds and flowers release red
pigment called hypercin,
which is photoreactive.

Preparations
Infused oils, tea from dried
leaves, tinctures

St. John's Wort Oil

The herbalist who lived in our home before us planted St. John's wort from seed throughout the front yard. It has since spread and naturalized there. Beginning around the summer solstice, after the morning dew I pick the fresh blooms and the bigger buds for this fresh oil. The finished oil is a deep ruby-red color.

At least 1 cup of fresh St. John's wort flowers and larger buds

Carrier oil of your choice (I usually use olive oil)

Pack the fresh flowers and buds into a clean glass jar. My St. John's wort comes in spurts, so I will often make a little at a time, then add more blooms and more oil as they come. Cover them with carrier oil and let sit in a warm and sunny place. This oil can only be made with fresh blooms, so I like to check on this infusion often to make sure no mold is forming, as fresh flowers contain more water. Shake once daily. Let sit for 4 to 6 weeks, or until the infusion has turned a dark red. Strain through a sieve lined with cheesecloth into a clean jar. I use the oil straight to rub on my neck or turn it into a salve (see page 289).

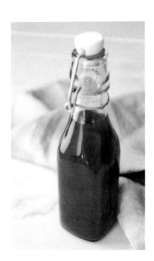

Tulsi

OCIMUM TENUIFLORUM

*T*ulsi is a sacred plant of Ayurveda and Indian culture that is cultivated in temples and many homes, where the act of tending the plant is a sacred ritual. Many species of basils are prized plants across many cultures. Tulsi grows well in our garden; like other basils, it enjoys full sun and being well watered. Tulsi is an adaptogen, supporting the body's responses to stressors and balancing and reducing the negative effects of stress on both physical and emotional health.

Tulsi is one of my favorite plants. A member of the basil family, it is easy to grow. Tulsi is an adaptogen, and its daily use helps fortify our nervous system to outside stressors. When I drink a cup of tulsi tea daily, I find stressors that normally make me feel off-kilter don't hit quite so deep. My capacity to handle the unpaid bill or the cries of my children grows. I am grounded, my nervous system is regulated, and I can handle more.

It is a fortifying ally during uncertain times and an all-around plant for supporting the body's immune system. Tulsi works in one way by keeping excess adrenaline and cortisol from being produced, increasing dopamine and serotonin levels, and promoting a calm focus. Tulsi can also aid cognitive performance, as it helps with cerebral circulation. In addition, it kindles digestive systems, clears the head and lungs, and is indicated for colds and congestions and stuck conditions.

You can make a tincture of the fresh flowering tops.

CAUTION: As tulsi may interfere with blood glucose, people with diabetes should take it only under the guidance of a health-care professional. Tulsi may temporarily reduce sperm count and sperm motility (Gardner and McGuffin, 2013).

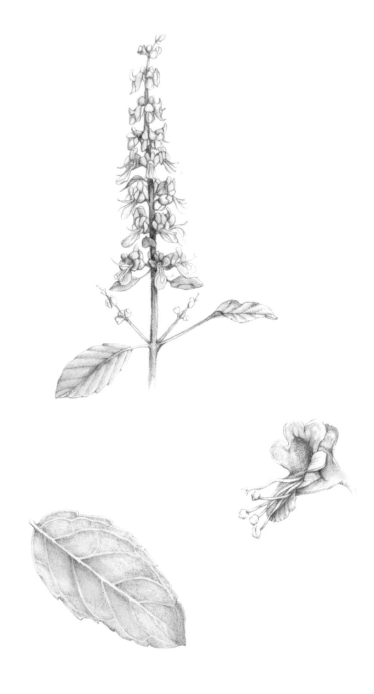

Plant family
Lamiaceae

Other names
Holy basil, sacred basil (India, where it is revered as a sacred plant)

Herbal actions
Adaptogen, alterative, anticancer, antidepressant, antimicrobial, antioxidant, antispasmodic, cardiotonic, carminative, diaphoretic, emmenagogue, expectorant, immunomodulant, nervine, radioprotective

---

Energetics
Warming and drying

Gather
Harvest leaves and flowers; when they bloom, I cut tops at the apical growth to encourage the plant to bush out.

Grow
Perennial only in tropical climates of USDA Hardiness Zone 10; grows as an annual in other zones. Suitable in a pot and in the garden beds; harvest as the plant begins to bloom. Seeds require light for germination so cover lightly with soil. Start seeds indoors 6 weeks before the last frost, then plant seedlings outside 2 feet apart.

Region
Grows wild in India, Sri Lanka, Pakistan, Bangladesh, southern China, Thailand, and Malaysia; can be grown in most temperate gardens

Flower essence
Opens heart and brow chakras; provides illumination around our heart's true purpose

---

Botanical description
An annual shrub that grows up to 2 feet, with hairy stems and oval, serrated leaves. Leaves range from light green to darker purple, with white to light purple tubular flowers.

Preparations
Can be used orally and topically in infused wine, teas, infused oils, smoothies, and infused into desserts

Holy Basil Sangria

Makes 4 servings

In a 1 liter glass jar, combine the fresh holy basil and white wine. Cover with a lid and refrigerate for at least 1 hour up to 4 hours. In a 1 liter pitcher, macerate the fruit and honey for 20 to 60 minutes. Strain the infused wine through a mesh strainer and pour it over the macerated fruit, gently stir in the brandy, and refrigerate for up to 4 hours. Serve over ice or sparkling water (if desired).

4 or 5 fresh flowering
holy basil or tulsi stems

1 (750 ml) bottle organic
white wine

1 cup fresh raspberries,
blackberries, or strawberries,
quartered

3 tablespoons honey

⅓ cup brandy
or Grand Marnier

Sparkling water, for serving
(optional)

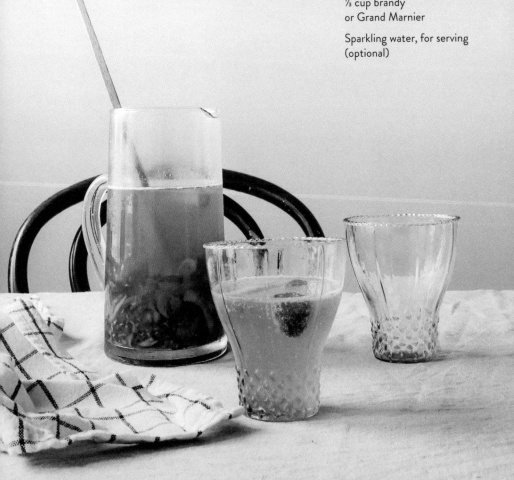

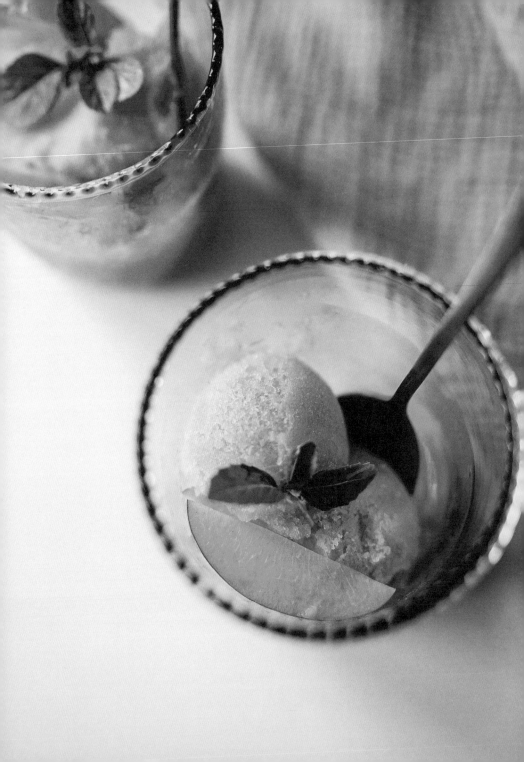

Tulsi and Peach Sorbet

Juicy ripe peaches and the unique flavor of holy basil come together to make this sorbet a summer favorite—a match made in seasonal heaven. It's also a delicious flavor combination for a shrub.

2 pounds ripe peaches

5 tablespoons freshly squeezed lemon juice

1 teaspoon almond extract or vanilla extract

1 tablespoon vodka

⅓ cup honey

1 cup holy basil or tulsi leaves, roughly chopped

Makes 4 to 6 servings

Prepare a bowl of ice water and set aside. Fill a large pot or Dutch oven with water and bring it to a boil. In batches, blanch the peaches, placing them in boiling water for 20 to 30 seconds, and then remove them with a slotted spoon to the ice water bath. Peel and pit the peaches, place the flesh in a blender or food processor along with the lemon juice, extract, and vodka. Puree for a minute, until smooth, cover, and refrigerate.

Combine 1 cup water, the honey, and tulsi in a large saucepan and bring to a boil over medium heat. Lower the heat to low and simmer for 10 minutes, stirring occasionally, until the honey is dissolved and the mixture is fragrant. Remove from the heat and let cool.

In a food processor, blend the honey tulsi syrup and peach puree. Transfer to an ice cream maker and follow the manufacturer's instructions, then transfer the mixture to a freezer-safe bowl or dish quickly before it begins to melt. Freeze for at least 1 hour, until ready to serve.

Yarrow ACHILLEA MILLEFOLIUM

A herbaceous flowering perennial, yarrow can be found in gardens, meadows, and prairies; it will naturalize in full sun and sandy soils. Yarrow can tolerate drought and heat, making it a wonderful addition to gardens in drought-prone locales. Yarrow helps with air pollution through capturing particulates in its leaves, and its flowers are a favorite of native pollinators. Collect seeds in late summer and early fall when the flowers' colors have faded to light tan.

Yarrow has always spoken to me about containers and boundaries—it's used to stop bleeding and is known for its wound healing properties and ability to break fevers. In the garden, yarrow balances the soil and deters pests. My children know yarrow is a good friend. The doctrine of signatures is evident in the leaves, as the feathery leaves indicate its uses for the blood vessels or capillaries.

Yarrow is used on swellings and mosquito bites by the Ho-Chunk people (Davis, 2010), and fresh leaves rubbed on the bite bring quick relief, as they do placed in the ear canal to treat earaches. With its antimicrobial effects, it's an ally for colds best taken in tea form for its diaphoretic properties that help open pores and stimulate sweating to bring down fevers. Dried and powdered yarrow works as an instant bandage on skinned knees and bleeding cuts and is a must-have in our first aid kit. It can also be made into a spit poultice for immediate relief to stop bleeding. In tincture form, yarrow has a tonifying effect on the uterus, balancing heavy menstruation and helping relieve spasms and cramps.

Yarrow flower essence and its spirit medicine aids us in cultivating personal and energetic boundaries. It's energetic medicine floods in when simply sitting in open awareness with a yarrow plant. Burning in herbal smoke can uplift your awareness and clear negative energy. Whether you need boundaries in toxic or codependent relationships or the noise of the outside world drowns out your own voice, yarrow helps knit together holes in the energetic field, so your energy is yours, not to be drained by others nor overflow into others.

CAUTION: Do not use yarrow during pregnancy.

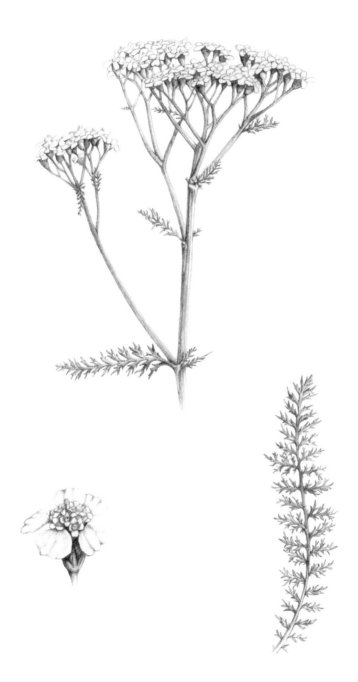

Plant family
Asteraceae

Other names
Hoocąk (Ho-Chunk),
translated a woodchuck tail

Region
Europe, North America,
western Asia

Botanical description
Green feathery alternate
leaves, almost fernlike,
branching only near the top.
Tiny white flowers with four
to six ray petals arranged in a
flat-topped cluster. Can grow
up to 3 feet tall when
flowering.

Grow
USDA Hardiness Zones 3 to
9. In cold weather climates,
sow seeds indoors 8 to 10
weeks before last frost; light
is required for germination.
Plant out after last frost in
full sun. Do not disturb
seedlings; water from the
bottom. Yarrow blooms 120
days after planting.

Gather
Aerial part: flowers and leaves
from May to October

Herbal actions
Anti-inflammatory,
antimicrobial, antispasmodic,
astringent, diaphoretic,
emmenagogue, vulnerary

Energetics
Cooling

Flower essence
For sensitive beings who are
easily influenced by their
environment and feel easily
depleted

Preparations
Tea, tincture, infused oil,
poultice

Bug Spray

Yarrow's volatile oils are known to repel mosquitos, ticks, and other insects; even planting yarrow in the garden can deter these pests. Those compounds are best extracted using tincture made from fresh yarrow plants. If insects are heavy, reapply this spray every 30 minutes or so; if not, a couple hours between applications should suffice.

A note on essential oils: Essential oils are made from the volatile oils in a plant, and they deter animals and bugs because of their potency. They are very concentrated and should be used sparingly, especially in products that will be going on the skin—never use them internally. In addition to the ones suggested here, other insect repellent essential oils include citronella, lemon eucalyptus, clove, and lemongrass.

1 part Yarrow Tincture (page 208)

1 part witch hazel

10 drops thyme essential oil

10 drops rosemary essential oil

15 drops lavender essential oil

10 drops tea tree essential oil

Special equipment: bottle with a spray top

Combine all the ingredients in a spray bottle and apply liberally to keep the bugs away in the summer months.

Seasonal Rhythms: Yarrow Three Ways

Powdered Yarrow

Harvest yarrow, both leaves and flowers, and hang upside down to dry or lay it flat on a screen. You will know it is dry when the plant becomes crispy between your fingers. In either a mortar or pestle or spice grinder, grind all the leaves, flowers, and stems into a powder and place in a clean jar. Use a pinch of dried yarrow on cuts and scrapes to stop the bleeding; almost instantly, yarrow creates a barrier and helps stop bleeding.

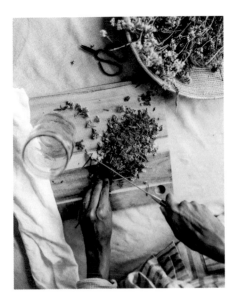

Yarrow Tincture: Folk Method

Fill a clean, sterilized quart-size jar with chopped fresh yarrow or dried yarrow, if you don't have access to fresh plant material; use half the amount if using dried herb, with a ratio of 1 part dried herb to 5 parts vodka or a ratio of 1 part fresh plant material to 3 parts vodka. Pour high-proof alcohol, vodka, or brandy over the chopped herbs until they are covered. Set in a dark pantry or cupboard for a full lunar cycle, new moon to new moon, about 4 weeks. Shake the jar every few days, imbuing it with your healing intention and energy. Strain through a metal sieve lined with organic muslin cloth and press on the herb, squeezing out all the liquid. Pour the tincture into amber dropper bottles and store, labeled with the herb and menstruum (solvent) used and the dates it was made and strained. Compost the leftover plant material.

Yarrow-Infused Oil: Alcohol Intermediary Method

This is one way of making a potent herbal oil that does not use a folk method. Feel free to use other herbs in this recipe or long folk method to make a yarrow oil. This demonstrates that there are many ways to make herbal preparations.

1 ounce dried yarrow

½ to 1 ounce 190-proof alcohol

8 ounces carrier oil

Makes 8 ounces

Grind the yarrow to a powder in a spice grinder and mix it in a pint jar with ½ ounce alcohol. Blend until the mixture is damp but not wet. Once the herbs and alcohol are combined, place a piece of parchment over the glass jar and close the lid. Let sit at room temperature for 24 hours.

Transfer the herb mixture to a blender with the carrier oil. Blend on medium speed until the blender feels warm to the touch and mixture is well blended, about 5 minutes. Transfer the mixture to a double boiler and heat over low for 1 hour. Strain the mixture through a fine-mesh strainer lined with organic muslin cloth and a widemouthed funnel. You may need to strain it a couple times to remove all the powdered herbs. Squeeze the cheesecloth to press out as much oil as possible. Bottle the oil in an amber bottle and label as described above.

Late Summer Herbal Smoke Bundles

This "recipe" involves a bundle of herbs, wrapped and dried together, to purify and cleanse a space for ceremonial and ritual practice. Often referred to as "smudging," it is a Native American spiritual and cultural ceremony. There is a conversation about the cultural appropriation and commercial exploitation of burning sacred plants such as palo santo and white sage, which have significance to other communities and cultures. These plants hold deep spiritual meaning and cultural references that are lost when brought to global markets. These plants are now being exploited, commodified, overharvested, and sold without the context or reverence to the plants. However, herbal cleansing or smudging spans many cultures and is used worldwide. We can decolonize our understanding and reclaim these ancestral practices by interacting with plants holding meaning to us. Herbal smoke is an important part of clearing the energy in our bodies and homes, and we can achieve potent healing from using herbs that are gathered or grown in our own bioregion, cultivating a personal relationship with the plant and participating in sacred ritual. Herbal smoke can help calm your energy and bring you back to center. Our wishes, dreams, and intentions are carried on smoke to our ancestors' ears.

These herbs are commonly used for herbal smoke bundles: rosemary for cleansing, juniper for abundance, yarrow for boundaries, white pine for trusting inner knowing, lavender for calming, prairie sage for purification, mugwort for dreaming and divination, and the mint family, like catnip, and bay leaves for protection.

Fresh plant cuttings

Undyed hemp or organic cotton twine

Gather your herbs with intention and reverence. Take only what you require, giving a little offering or asking permission. Using shears, clip what you need. Let the plants wilt in a harvesting basket or on a screen for a day before bundling them. Evergreens can be wrapped immediately, but be sure to wrap them tightly, as they will shrink while they dry.

With twine (remember to use something without chemicals as you will be burning the thread, too), tie the bundle together tightly about an inch from the base, leaving a few inches extra. Tightly wrap the twine and string around the bundle as you move up, keeping the plant material clasped tightly together. Wrap the string around the top of the bundle and make your way back down, straightening it as you go. Meeting at the beginning, wrap the string around the base again, securing it in a double knot with the extra string at the base. Trim the ends. Hang the bundle away from light and dry until the herbs are crispy, a few weeks and up to a month for evergreens.

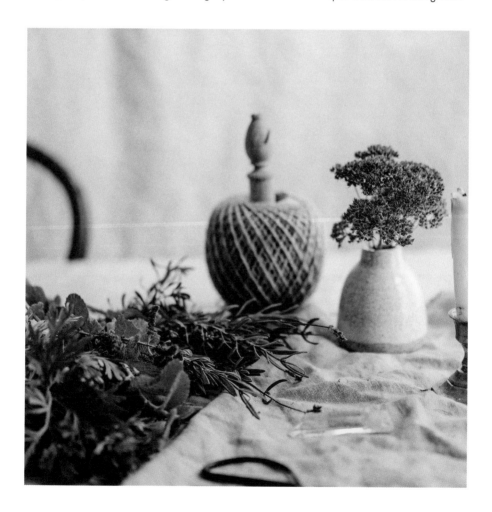

Autumn

Seasonal Rhythms

The verdant green of summer drains from the
foliage to reveal shades of amber and gold.

Waning
Crescent Moon

Autumn Equinox
Around September 22

Astrology of autumn
Libra (cardinal air), Scorpio (fixed water),
Sagittarius (mutable fire)

Downward
Energy

Energetics of autumn
Dry becoming cold

Element
Earth

The West,
Sunset

GATHER: Seeds, the last flowers
and fruits of the season; dig
elecampane, burdock, and dandelion.

MAKE: Use whatever culinary
herbs are left in the garden to make
an herbal equinox wreath with dried
flowers and herbal posies to gift to
friends and family.

DO: Visit an apple orchard, cry,
host a harvest meal, make bonfires
to watch the full moon. Slow cook
pots of bone broth on the stovetop.
Honor those lost to violence,
injustice, and oppression.

In September, we harvest fruit, root, and seed from the plants, and the energy descends back into the roots for regeneration. The autumn equinox, a day of balance, forewarns a shift in the light. Purple asters awaken on the prairie, signaling summer's decline. Change is in the air. There is an urgency to soak every moment of warmth, of green, and squirrel it away. The bright Harvest or full Corn Moon's light glows bright so farmers can harvest crops deep into the night. Dance, sing, howl at the moon. Elderberries ripen; gather them before the birds do. This is a season of gratitude and abundance, change and transition.

Wet, damp autumn rains chill to the bone. Golden leaves fall willingly from the trees or are stripped by strong winds. Skeletons of Queen Anne's lace dance with morning dew across the meadow; sleepy goldenrod, drained of its luster, goes to seed. Autumn is an embodiment of grief, of harvesting what has been sown, of preparing the soil and body for rest. The season to harvest roots, we likewise return to our roots. Like the plants' energy returning to their root systems to conserve energy and wait in hibernation until the sun returns, our bodies begin to hibernate. We move less to conserve our energy. Cultural celebrations across the Earth turn to remembrance of our dead. Remembering our ancestors as the roots from which our lives arose. In recalling their names on our breath, it keeps them alive in our hearts, dancing alive in our bones, cooking their favorite foods, their spirit lives in us. In the slowdown of this season, we can begin to process the events throughout the year. Our bodies crave warmth and connection with community.

October is a time of preparation and transformation. Cleaning up the garden beds, gathering seeds, preparing and nourishing the soil with cover crops, raked leaves, or fresh compost, we save our soil from extinction. Give back to the earth for all it gives to you. Press your hands in the soil in thanks for the harvest, connect. We prepare what we've grown and celebrate with a harvest dinner, preparing our hearts and minds for the long term: winter.

Fall is a liminal season, a passageway between life and death. Death envelops us; as plants die back you can smell decay in the air. Now is time to dig trenches for spring bulbs in somatic practice of hope and make our preparations for the long nights to come. Cold and flu season is upon us. Making warming and nourishing meals helps support the immune system. Darkness comes earlier each evening; it grows colder. Dinner by candlelight; gaze into the wood fire in the hearth or bonfires outside as the full Beaver Moon or Frost Moon rises in the crisp twilight air. I nourish myself in solitude and reestablish my boundaries.

Seed Keeping:
A Season of Gratitude

Collecting, threshing, winnowing, and saving seeds is an act of service to the land. A seed is the end of the life of a plant yet contains all information necessary for new life. A mirror of the cyclical nature of all life, of living, death, and rebirth, contained within our cells.

We harvest and keep the grain of information and knowledge for the season ahead and cherish gifts from the earth for survival. Saving seeds is about preserving our history, genetic diversity, and sovereignty over our food. My African ancestors braided sacred seeds into their hair for safe keeping, all the genetic knowledge carried within a microscopic space. Humans have practiced saving seeds for centuries. When we save seeds from the plants grown in our area, it encourages adaptation to climate shifts, and it cultivates a deep relationship with the food we eat and our environment. When done on a larger community scale, the practice cultivates resilience, strengthens our food systems as we are sharing seeds adapted to the local ecosystem and climate. I often collect, save, dry, and share seeds from my calendula, peas, flowers, tomatoes, dill, cilantro, ground cherries, and pumpkins, although squash are more prone to cross-pollination. Saving seeds is a sacred ritual; Indigenous communities around the world continue this tradition as stewards of their land and biodiversity.

I learned a few tips about saving seeds from a local Amish woman at our farmers' market: For tomatoes or ground cherries, for instance, wait until the plant is fully ripe, scoop out the seeds into a jar of water, and leave them until the seeds have sunk to the bottom. Pour away the liquid and leave the seeds to dry on a cloth. Once they are fully dry, place them in an envelope or airtight container. Label them with the date, the name, the variety, and the garden they came from. In winter, host a local seed swap to share seeds with neighbors and friends. This is how community grows stronger.

Apple MALUS DOMESTICA

*A*pple is a medicine all its own. It takes an apple tree from four to six years to bear its fruits. Since it produces its fruits in autumn, I think of apple as Virgo medicine. Like strawberries, raspberries, blackberries, peaches, pears, and roses, apples—our most beloved fruit—come from the rose family. Apples are filled with vitamins and minerals, such as vitamins A and C, beta carotene, dietary fiber, and calcium. With its bright red color and shape, the doctrine of signatures indicates apples are for the heart.

Apples have the proven ability to reduce the risk of chronic diseases and support a healthy immune system while balancing blood sugar and helping lower cholesterol and risk of diabetes. The fiber in apple pectin helps regulate the digestive systems, both soothing diarrhea and acting as a laxative. Pectin is astringent and can be used for wounds. Apple cider vinegar is supportive of the immune system and digestion and is the base of many herbal medicines; it can also be used as a substitute for alcohol in extracting the medicinal qualities of plants, making it cost-effective and safe for those with sensitivities to alcohol.

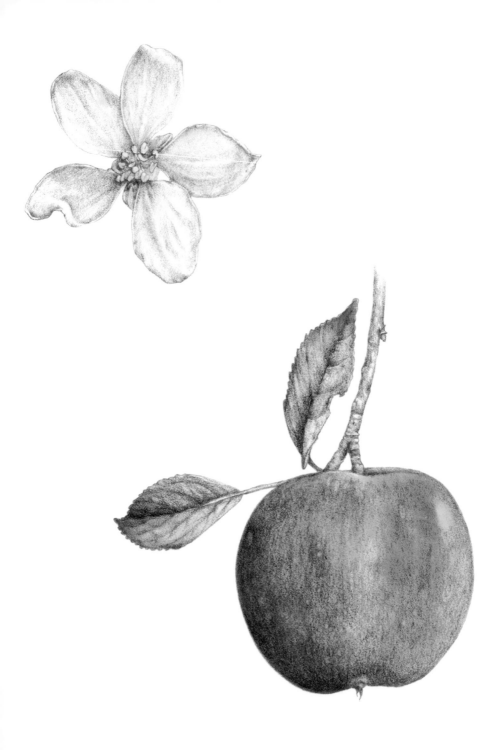

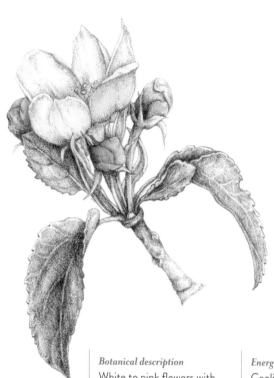

Plant family
Rosaceae

Other names
Linch'in (Chinese)

Region
Native to temperate regions in both the Northern and Southern Hemispheres, modern day varieties developed in Europe and North America

Botanical description
White to pink flowers with five petals blooming in May, ripening into a round, flesh, and edible fruit. Leaves have finely toothed edges.

Gather
Apple blossoms turn to fruit in September, about three to six months after blooms appear.

Herbal actions
Antibacterial, anti-inflammatory, antiviral, astringent, diuretic, tonic

Energetics
Cooling, moist, sweet

Flower essence
Apple flower essence imparts clarity and purifies the body of past woes. It helps one care and tend for the body with nourishing thoughts, habits, and actions and embrace one's imperfections.

Preparations
Eaten raw for the most benefit, apples can be turned into cooked desserts, cider, and vinegars, and stewed.

Herbal Spiced Apple Cider

This recipe brings two rose family favorites into a
heartwarming blend. Paired with carminative spices, this
homemade cider recipe takes a little more time and patience,
but that is what heart medicine teaches us: the sweetness in
life is worth the work and worth the wait. Apple and hawthorn
impart softness and strength for our journeys, and I love to
share this recipe with friends and family throughout autumn.
As the seasons shift and as we hold grief in our hearts for what
is passing, this cider helps us soften into our heart space.

6 cups fresh apple cider

2 cinnamon sticks

3 whole star anise

1 thumb-size piece fresh
ginger, peeled and sliced

3 orange slices and/
or 3 strips of orange peel

1 tablespoon whole cloves

2 teaspoons cardamom pods

2 tablespoons dried
hawthorn berries

⅓ cup of honey, or to taste

1 bay leaf

*Makes
4 to 6
servings*

Combine all the ingredients in a Dutch oven,
over medium heat. Leaving the pot uncovered,
bring the mixture to a simmer—be careful not to
let it come to a full boil. Adjust the heat to maintain
a very low simmer, cover, and cook for about 30 minutes.
Remove from the heat and let cool a bit before straining the
mixture through cheesecloth, pressing to remove as much of
the juices as possible. Compost the fruit pulp and spices.

Store the cider in the refrigerator for up to a week. Reheat
if you'd like to serve it warm with a cinnamon stick, an apple
slice, or a splash of brandy for a holiday party.

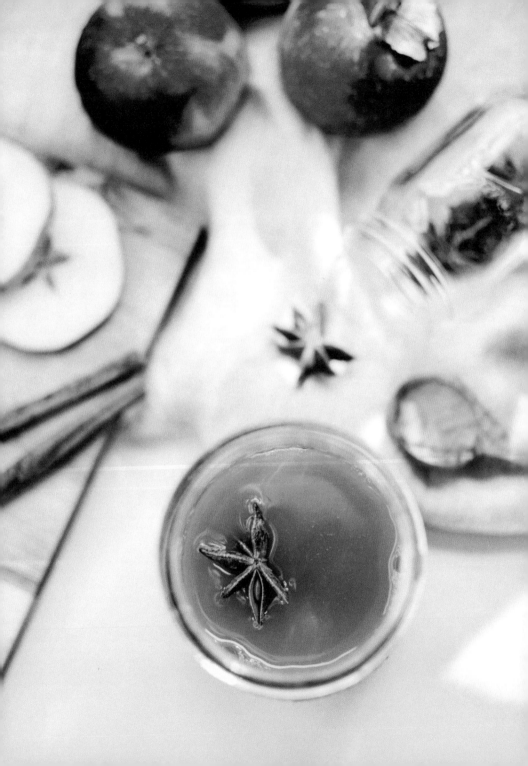

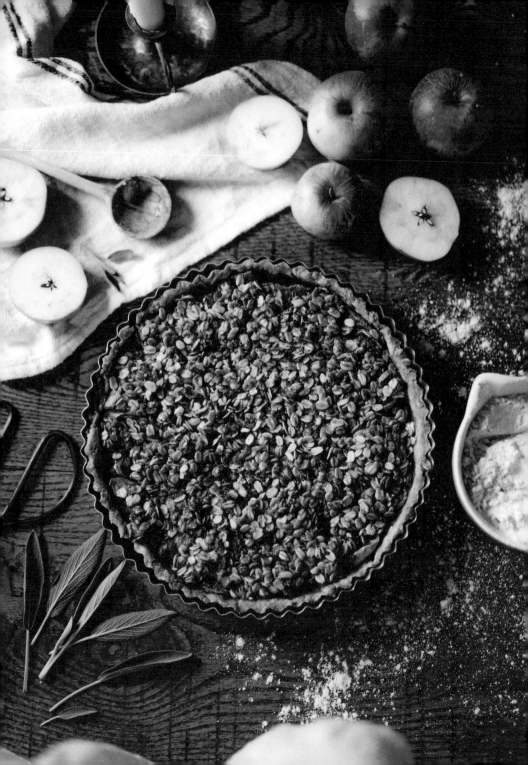

Apple and Sage Crumble

You can use this as filling in a piecrust (see page 260) or make it in a baking dish.

Makes 8 servings

Place the apples in a large bowl, mix in ¼ cup of the honey, the cinnamon, cardamom, vanilla extract, and ⅛ teaspoon salt until coated. Transfer to a large skillet and cook over low to medium heat until the apples have softened and have taken on a caramel color, about 8 minutes. Remove the skillet from the heat, stir in lemon zest and juice and the chopped sage leaves. Pour into a greased baking dish or prepared pie crust.

Using a pastry cutter, combine the cold butter cubes, the remaining ¼ honey, ⅛ teaspoon salt, sage chiffonade, and flour in a mixing bowl. Once the ingredients are combined and the pieces of butter are pea-size, stir in the rolled oats. Sprinkle evenly over the apples, covering the fruit completely.

Place the baking dish in the oven and bake for 30 to 40 minutes, until bubbling and browned. Serve with vanilla ice cream.

5 large apples (about 3 pounds), cored and chopped

½ cup honey

½ teaspoon ground cinnamon

¼ teaspoon ground cardamom

1 teaspoon vanilla extract

¼ teaspoon salt

2 or 3 fresh sage leaves, chopped, plus 10 to 12 sage leaves cut into a chiffonade

Zest and juice of ½ lemon

5 tablespoons unsalted butter

¾ cup flour (wheat or almond)

1½ cups rolled oats

Vanilla ice cream, for serving

Beet BETA VULGARIS

Beets are seen as a blood-cleansing food, especially in Haitian culture. Beets are root chakra medicine at its finest, exemplifying a strong doctrine of signatures: their deep red juices, growing as a literal root in the ground. Beets are a tonic and nutritive food and contain blood-building minerals, including iron, zinc, magnesium, potassium, calcium, vitamins C and B6, and folate. Its nutrition and carotenoids act to support the body's nervous system. Beets are effective in lowering blood pressure, which supports cardiovascular health. Beet root can be used as a natural food coloring. Beets help us feel nourished and grounded—rooted—so we can fully embrace our lives and potential.

Plant family
Amaranthaceae

Region
Grows wild along the coastlines of North Africa, Asia, and Europe; cultivated around the world

Botanical description
The root is a deep red, round bulb; beets are biennial plants that flower in the second year.

Grow
Beets are a simple and easy vegetable to grow. Sow seeds ½ inch deep and 1 inch apart in early spring before the last frost and in late summer 4 to 6 weeks before first frost for a fall harvest. Germinate in 7 days.

Gather
Harvest and prepare both roots and leaves.

Herbal actions
Carminative, tonic

Energetics
Warming, aromatic, sweet

Flower essence
Transmuting trauma of the root chakra; rebalances our root to remember the sweetness of life; land healing, ancestral trauma, and helping us trust

Preparations
Prepared raw or cooked, juiced, powdered, roasted, or fermented. Leaves can be used in pesto or to replace spinach in recipes.

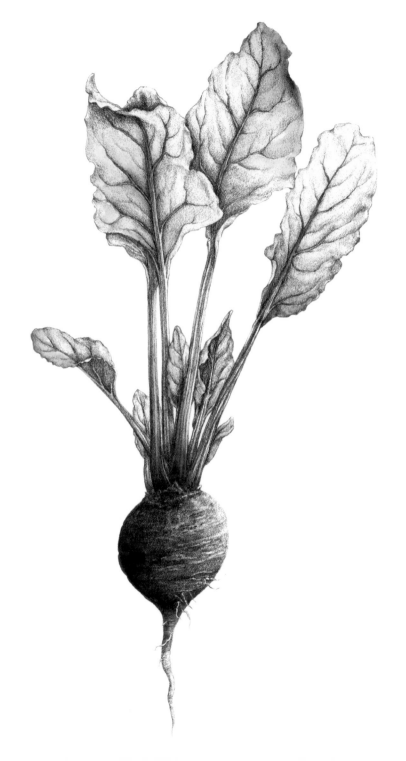

Beet and Burdock Sauerkraut

In African American traditions, beet roots and their juice are used as a blood cleanser. Beets are known to lower blood pressure and strengthen the nervous system. This kraut is packed with nutrients and herbs to support a healthy gut and root.

1 small red cabbage, shredded (about 3 cups)

2 tablespoons kosher salt, plus more if needed

2 raw medium beets, julienned (about 1 cup)

1 medium apple, cored and shredded (about ¼ cup)

1-inch piece fresh ginger, peeled and grated

3 garlic cloves, minced

2 burdock roots

2 teaspoons fennel seeds

Makes 1 quart jar

Start by sanitizing your hands, sterilizing utensils and a quart jar.

Place the shredded cabbage in a large bowl and add the salt. Using your clean hands, massage the cabbage until it breaks down and becomes soft, about 3 minutes. Cover the bowl with a kitchen towel and let sit 10 minutes as it breaks down further and releases its juices.

Add the julienned beets, massage with your hands, cover, and let sit for another 2 minutes. Then mix in the shredded apple, ginger, garlic, and burdock until combined. Add the fennel seeds. Transfer the mixture to a jar, packing everything tightly and pushing the mixture all the way down until it's submerged in its own juices. Leave 1½ inches of headspace at the top of the jar. If there is not enough brine, you can dissolve 1 teaspoon kosher sea salt in 1 cup water and add it to the jar. Place a weight on the shredded mixture and cover the jar with a cloth or fermentation lid. Culture at room temperature for at least 3 days minimum and up to 7 (typically, 4 or 5 days is good), then refrigerate.

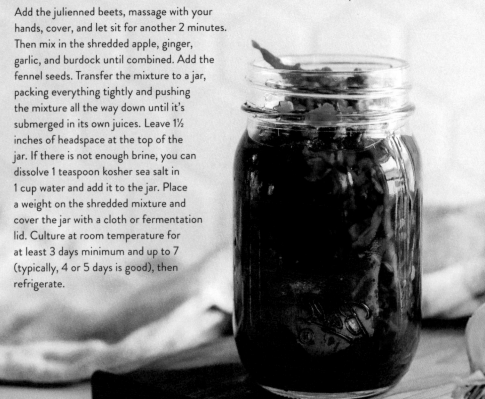

Burdock ARCTIUM LAPPA

A common weed, burdock has been used throughout the world as a source of food, from European and African American to Indigenous American materia medica. Burdock is one of the most important detoxifying herbs in Western and Chinese medicine. Burdock's often six-foot-deep roots help cleanse and remove toxins in fevers and infections and move the body into a state of health. Most effective when used over a longer period of time, it can be incorporated into food in many ways.

The fresh leaves can be used crushed as a poultice on cuts and bruises. I like to incorporate burdock into broths. It has inulin, a type of fiber that serves as a prebiotic for digestion. Burdock works from the inside out, clearing skin conditions such as eczema and psoriasis. The action for removing waste products helps clear chronic skin conditions and cleanse the blood. I mix burdock with dandelion and yellow dock in the Spring Cleansing Tonic (page 99).

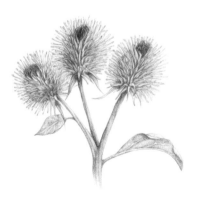

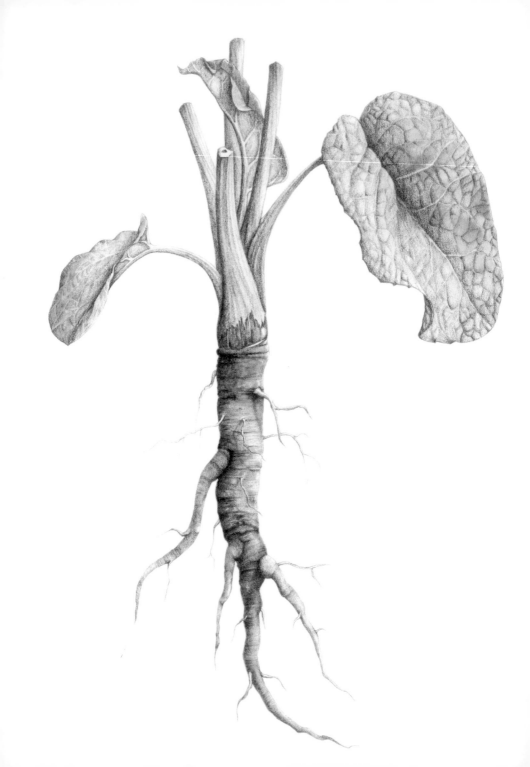

Plant family
Asteraceae

Other names
Lappa, beggar's button

Region
Native to Europe and Asia; grows in temperate regions worldwide

---

Botanical description
Triangular leaf rosettes in the first year with a taproot. It has pink or purple thistle flowers in the second year. The burdock taproot has white inner flesh and is large and fibrous and can extend 6 feet down.

Parts used
Roots and rhizome

Gather
Dig roots and rhizome of first-year plants in spring or fall; roots may loosen from the ground after a rain.

Herbal actions
Alterative, analgesic, anti-inflammatory, antioxidant, bitter, diaphoretic, diuretic, laxative, nutritive, tonic, vulnerary

---

Energetics
Bitter, moistening and cooling

Flower essence
Caught up in deep old anger

Preparations
Decoction, tincture, pickled, in soups and stews

Burdock Bitters

Bitters are made similarly to a tincture. With modern societies' prevalence and craving for sweet and salty, bitter tastes can be hard to come by, but they are so necessary in the digestive process. Wild and foraged plants are an antidote. They can be taken on the tongue or added to sparkling water, ginger ale, or a cocktail. They aid in increasing the digestive enzymes and bile production through the mechanism of bitter taste on the tongue, increasing saliva. Dandelion and burdock are a common and well-loved combination for bitters.

½ cup chopped fresh dandelion root, or ¼ cup dried

½ cup chopped fresh burdock root, or ¼ cup dried

2 teaspoons sliced fresh ginger

1 tablespoon fresh or dried orange peel

5 cardamom pods

2 cups organic vodka or brandy

Makes 1 pint jar

In a clean quart-size jar, combine all the ingredients. Cover the jar with a lid and label it with the ingredients and date. Place the jar in a cool dark place for 4 weeks or a full moon cycle, new moon to new moon or full moon to full moon, shaking it very well every few days. After 4 weeks, strain the mixture through a fine mesh strainer, pressing on the herbs to extract as much flavor and liquid as possible. Label and store the bitters in a cool place or the refrigerator for up to a year. To use, place 15 drops on your tongue or add up to 1 ounce to sparkling water or a cocktail before or after a meal to aid with digestive function. You can divide it among dropper bottles to give as gifts to friends.

Elderberry SAMBUCUS CANADENSIS

*E*lderberries are the ripe fruit of the elderflower. Growing in hedgerows and under scrub in the woods and along roadsides, elderberries are used for protection and purification. When prepared correctly, elderberries help alleviate cold and flu symptoms. Elderberries should not be consumed raw. The raw plant contains cyanogenic glycosides and can be toxic. With the flowers harvested at summer's edge and berries in the autumn, it stands between two worlds.

Elderberry was the first herbal preparation I made before my garden birthed me into an herbalist. In my city kitchen, I gathered dried berries from a jar, honey for sweetness, and my trusted kitchen spices, cinnamon stick and clove. It was my second cold and flu season as a mother, and a friend had shared her experience making elderberry syrup for her little one. Standing over the bubbling and boiling pot, I stirred casting spells and thought of my elders undertaking the same to keep their babies well.

Because of its antiviral and immune-stimulant actions, elderberry taken at the onset of symptoms can reduce the duration of the cold or flu, as it interferes with the virus replication. European elderberries (*Sambucus nigra*) are larger and have a darker purple color when ripe than American elder (*S. canadensis*).

CAUTION: Red elderberry (*Sambucus racemosa*), with bright red fruit, is poisonous. Elderberries appear similar to the more toxic pokeberry, but pokeberry is not arranged on an umbel like elderberry. Also be diligent in removing as much stem as possible from the elderberries, as the stems are mildly toxic and can cause nausea and diarrhea.

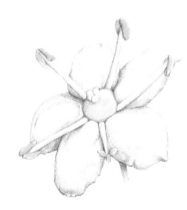

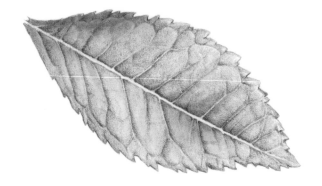

Plant family
Adoxaceae

Other names
Black elder, pipe tree

Region
Europe, Morocco, Algeria, western and central Asia. This variety is native to the Americas, east of the Rockies and south to Bolivia. There are other medicinal species distributed worldwide.

Botanical description
Leaves compound and opposite pairs, pinnate, five to nine leaflets; creamy white flowers with five petals in corymbs; fruit clusters of dark purple to black berries, 3 to 5 mm, on pink or green stems

Grow
USDA Hardiness Zones 3 to 9. Plant in hedgerows, wet and dry soils, prefers full sun. Can propagate from seed, root division, and cuttings. Take a cutting, using rooting hormone or cinnamon to prevent fungus, and place it in a jar of clean water for 2 months. Once the cutting grows roots, plant it in the garden. Elder also spreads through its taproot.

Gather
Berries are ready to harvest in late summer or early fall when they have turned from green to purple. Remove berries from the stems, because stems can be toxic.

Herbal actions
Anti-inflammatory, antioxidant, antiviral, immune stimulant

Energetics
Cooling

Preparations
Syrups, tea, jellies, tinctures

Elderberry Jelly

Makes 4
half-pint
jars

In a pot, bring 4 cups fresh elderberries and ¾ cup water to a simmer to release the juices. If you are using dried elderberries, use 2 cups of dried elderberries and 4 cups of water.

Remove the pot from the heat and pour the mixture through a muslin-lined sieve into a large measuring cup, compost the berries. If you don't have 4 cups of juice, top it off with another fruit juice (I like to add peach nectar). Pour the elderberry juice into a saucepan and bring to a boil over medium heat. Add the lemon juice, then stir in calcium water and reduce the heat to a simmer. In a small bowl, mix sweetener and pectin until blended, then stir it into the elderberry juice. Simmer.

Remove the saucepan from the heat and ladle the jelly into hot, sterilized pint-size canning jars, leaving ¼ inch of headspace, wipe down the rim with a damp cloth and cover with a clean lid and ring. Let cool at room temperature and then place the jelly in the fridge; alternatively, process the jars in a water bath for 10 minutes. The jelly will solidify as it cools.

4 cups fresh elderberries or 2 cups dried elderberries (to yield 4 cups elderberry juice)

1 ½ cups lemon juice

2 teaspoons calcium water

2 cups honey

2 teaspoons low-sugar pectin (I use Pomona's Universal Pectin)

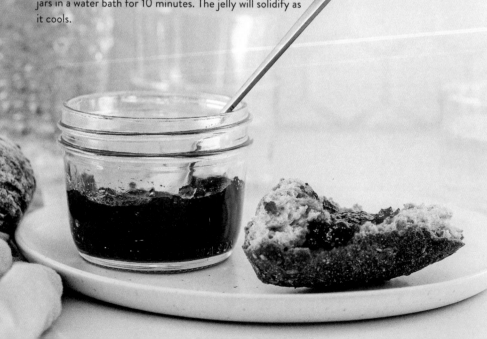

Elderberry Balsamic BBQ Sauce

½ cup Elderberry Jelly
(page 231)

½ cup ketchup

¼ cup balsamic vinegar

2 tablespoons
Worcestershire sauce

2 tablespoons Dijon mustard

4 teaspoons paprika

1 teaspoon minced garlic

1 teaspoon powdered ginger

2 tablespoons lemon juice

¼ teaspoon kosher salt

⅛ teaspoon ground cinnamon

In a saucepan over medium heat, combine all the ingredients
and bring to a simmer. Cook until the sauce thickens, about
15 minutes. Baste on meats during the last minutes of grilling.

Elderberry Syrup

*Elderberry syrup was one of the first home remedies I made
as a new mother. This is now a staple in our apothecary. Note
that this is thinner in consistency than store-bought syrups.*

Makes
1 quart
jar

Place the elderberries, cinnamon sticks,
cardamom pods, fresh ginger, citrus peel,
cloves, 4 cups water, and any add-ins (if using)
into a saucepan over medium heat. Bring the mixture
to a boil, then reduce heat to medium-low and simmer
until the liquid is reduced by half, anywhere from 30 to
60 minutes. As the berries begin to steam, mash them with a
fork or potato masher to release the juices. Remove the pan
from the heat and allow the elderberry juice to cool. Strain
the liquid through a fine-mesh sieve or cheesecloth and into a
pint jar; compost or discard the spent berries and spices. Add
honey to the liquid in the jar, shake to dissolve. When needed,
take 1 teaspoon up to three times daily. Store your elderberry
syrup in the refrigerator for up to 2 months.

1 cup fresh elderberries
(see Note), or ¾ cup dried

2 cinnamon sticks

3 whole cardamom pods

1 tablespoon sliced or grated
fresh ginger

Peel from a whole fresh
orange or lemon

6 dried whole cloves

1 cup honey

Optional add-ins:
1 tablespoon dried calendula,
1 tablespoon dried astragalus
root, 2 tablespoons fresh or
dried rose hips

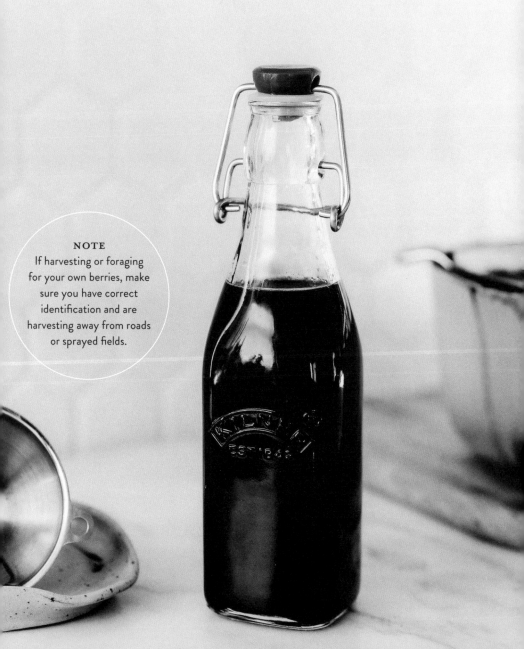

NOTE
If harvesting or foraging for your own berries, make sure you have correct identification and are harvesting away from roads or sprayed fields.

Elecampane INULA HELENIUM

A member of the sunflower family, elecampane prefers growing in damp earth. Its flowers bloom on sturdy hollow stocks of second-year plants, usually in July in our garden. Elecampane's large, fleshy root with a pungent aroma moves stuck mucus and is a tonic herb for the respiratory system, warming and cleaning. Elecampane can help us move those words, feelings, experiences we can't get off our chest or that are stuck in our throats. Elecampane unlocks grief and helps us release it.

Elecampane is high in inulin, a prebiotic fiber found in roots like dandelion and burdock, that is wonderful for moving along digestion and building a healthy immune system. Its mucilage helps soothe bronchial and stomach linings and is good for damp and cold conditions in the lungs. In traditional Chinese medicine, grief is stored in the lungs, and elecampane added to rose aids in healing and moving grief from our system. To decoct or concentrate it, simmer 1 teaspoon of root in 8 ounces of water over medium heat for 15 minutes.

CAUTION: Do not use elecampane during pregnancy or nursing. It is safe for young and old and often used in cases of chronic bronchitis and tuberculosis. Those with allergies to members of the Asteraceae family may find it also causes allergic reactions.

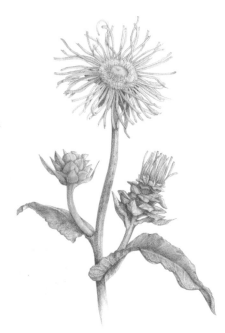

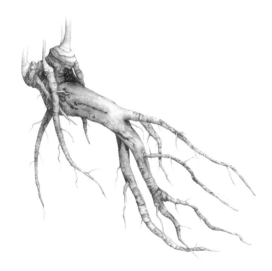

Plant family
Asteraceae

Other names
Wild sunflower, elfwort, xuan fu hua (TCM)

Region
Native to southeastern Europe and western Asia; grows in temperate regions throughout the United States; cultivated from seed

Botanical description
First year, a basal rosette of lance-shaped leaves; in the second year, a stalk perennial growing to 6 feet with yellow daisy-like flowers on a sturdy stem; oblong and alternate leaves. Roots are large, fleshy, brown on the outside, and white within.

Gather
The roots in the fall of its second or third year. Before this time, the plant is not ready, and after two years the root can become too woody. In the spring, before the aerial parts shoot up and in the fall after the plant has died back, dig roots, cut up and dry at a high temperature.

Herbal actions
Expectorant, antibacterial, antimicrobial, carminative, tonic, vermifuge, alterative

Energetics
Bitter and pungent, warming and drying

Flower essence
Stand in your power

Preparations
Tincture, honey, vinegar, syrup, decoction

Elecampane Honey

Stirred into a cup of hot water, lemon slices, and sliced fresh ginger, this is a wonderful concoction to support respiratory issues and stagnation in the lungs or digestive system, or when you need help moving grief.

¼ cup sliced elecampane root, fresh or dried

1 cup raw or local honey

Makes 1 cup

Fill a pint-size jar halfway with the sliced elecampane. Pour honey over the roots to cover and stir with a chopstick. Place a lid on the jar. Store the jar on a pantry shelf, shaking it daily. The honey is ready in one week. Strain and store in a sterilized pint jar in the cupboard.

NOTE
This infused honey can also be used in making the elecampane syrup recipe below.

Rose Hip and Elecampane Syrup

Elecampane is a wonderful remedy for congested coughs. It is great for breaking up mucus and congestion. Elecampane can be drying, which is why it pairs so well with rose hips, which are very high in vitamin C, in the syrup.

¼ cup dried elecampane root

¼ cup dried and chopped rose hips

2 teaspoons sliced fresh ginger

1 cinnamon stick

1 cup honey

Brandy (optional)

Makes 3 cups

Combine the elecampane, rose hips, ginger, and cinnamon stick, and 3 cups water in a covered saucepan and simmer for 25 to 35 minutes. Pour the mixture through a cheesecloth-lined strainer into a large measuring cup (you want an equal amount of liquid and honey, so measure it). Add the honey while the liquid is still warm to dissolve it. Add brandy, if using, as a preservative. Store the syrup in the refrigerator for up to a month. This syrup is wonderful for sore throats and wet coughs; take 2 teaspoons every 2 hours to relieve symptoms.

Garlic ALLIUM SATIVUM

*G*arlic is the epitome of food as medicine. Used worldwide as a base of cooking, it is a pungent and powerful herbal remedy for home and everyday use. Utilized for a variety of ailments, its pungent odor and taste fight infections and kill the growth of organisms like candida in the body's systems. Indicated for cholesterol, circulatory disorders, and high blood pressure, garlic moves the blood. Hung in homes from rafters and by the back door, garlic is seen in a spiritual sense as protective, warding off germs as well as negative energies and those who do us harm.

Garlic was commonly used in enslaved Africans' herbal repertoire as well as their cooking. Garlic is used to purify the blood and clear the root chakra, moving blocked energy, stuck emotions, and trauma. A strong antifungal, it can be used topically and internally to treat fungal infections. Garlic is used to expel worms and parasites and to treat respiratory infections. A garlic clove warmed in a cast-iron pan and placed gently in the ear can help with earaches, as it does infused in oil with mullein flowers.

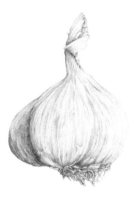

Plant family
Alliaceae

Other names
Da suan (TCM), rasoon (Ayurveda)

Region
Cultivated in the Middle East for 5,000 years; naturalized worldwide

Botanical description
Perennial herb related to the onion; grows erect with a flowering stem 2 to 3 feet in height. Light purple flowers; long, narrow, and flat leaves. White bulb of grouped cloves is covered in a papery skin.

Grow
Plant in the fall for a summer harvest. Separate out each head into cloves and space them 6 inches apart in loose, well-drained soil. Cover with a layer of fallen leaves or straw.

Gather
In late summer to early fall, bulbs can be dug, brushed off, and hung to dry.

Herbal actions
Antibiotic, expectorant, anti-diabetic, antiparasitic, antimicrobial, antiseptic, antiviral, carminative, antispasmodic, aphrodisiac, diaphoretic

Energetics
Warming, bitter

Flower essence
Brings wholeness, uniting the physical and spiritual body

Body systems affinities
Stomach, large intestine, circulatory

Preparations
Infused honey, infused oil, tincture, syrup, eaten raw for potency and used in salad dressings

Four Thieves Vinegar

Used as a salad dressing or a shot to ward off illness, "Four Thieves" is a well-known blend, comparable to fire cider. Paired with thyme, cinnamon, sage, cloves, rosemary, and ginger, this is a wonderful expectorant and antiviral recipe. I enjoy this as the base of salad dressings and marinades. As the story from French folklore goes, during an outbreak of the plague in the medieval period, a group of thieves were robbing the dead and their graves in Marseille, France. They covered their own bodies and faces in this herbal vinegar, and its strong antibacterial and antiviral properties protected them from catching the plague. Their secret recipe allowed them to commit the robberies without falling ill. When they were finally caught, they traded their secret recipe for leniency. Today, Four Thieves is used similarly to fight germs.

Some traditional recipes call for the addition of wormwood, juniper berries, horehound, angelica, and mint. Modern variations often contain the commonplace herbs and the spices included in this recipe, but feel free to experiment a bit.

1 to 2 tablespoons fresh rosemary

1 to 2 tablespoons fresh lavender

1 to 2 tablespoons fresh sage

1 to 2 tablespoons fresh thyme

2 or 3 cinnamon sticks

1 garlic clove

4 whole cloves

Peel of 1 lemon

16 ounces vinegar, such as organic apple cider, white wine, or champagne vinegar

Makes 2 cups

Combine all the ingredients in a 32-ounce glass jar. Cover the opening with a square of parchment, screw on the lid, and let this infuse for a week or two. I will decant, dilute with water, and transfer it into my spray bottle to clean kitchen counters and doorknobs in the winter season. When infused in culinary vinegar, it makes for delicious salad dressings and marinades.

Goldenrod SOLIDAGO RUGOSA

*B*looming on prairies, meadows, and fields in September, the perennial goldenrod signals corn is ripening. Goldenrod provides an important ecological function to native pollinators and honeybees. Goldenrod can be used to improve urinary health and dries out damp tissue states as it tones mucus membranes in the respiratory system. With its antimicrobial properties, it is used in Native American ethnobotany for burns and wound healing.

Use as a tea or tincture for clearing excess mucus in the sinuses, or as a tea for urinary tract inflammation, irritation, and kidney stones.

CAUTION: Goldenrod is not recommended for use in pregnant women or those with high blood pressure or hypertension. Do not use with pharmaceuticals for kidney issues. Proceed with caution as goldenrod has poisonous look-alikes, including a family called groundsel, staggerwort, and ragweed. If you are unsure of your find, leave it until you are confident.

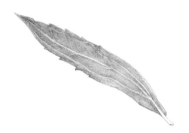

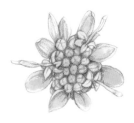

Plant family
Asteraceae

Region
USDA Hardiness Zones 4–8. Native to eastern and central regions of North America, southeast China, and parts of Europe. There are about 100 species worldwide.

Botanical descriptions
Narrow toothed leaves, thin sprays of small yellow flowers

Gather
Harvest the flowering tops in summer through fall just as they are starting to open for the most potent medicine. If you're drying, harvest when the flowers are budding to prevent the flowers from going to seed. Harvest leaves before the flowers open.

Herbal actions
Anti-inflammatory, astringent, antiseptic, carminative, decongestant, diaphoretic, diuretic

Energetics
Cooling, warming, stimulating, toning

Flower essence
Standing strong in oneself, an essence for perseverance. When you have trouble being true to yourself due to peer pressure or social demands, goldenrod brings you to center.

Body systems affinities
Respiratory and urinary tract systems

Preparations
Infused in white wine, tinctures, teas, infused oil

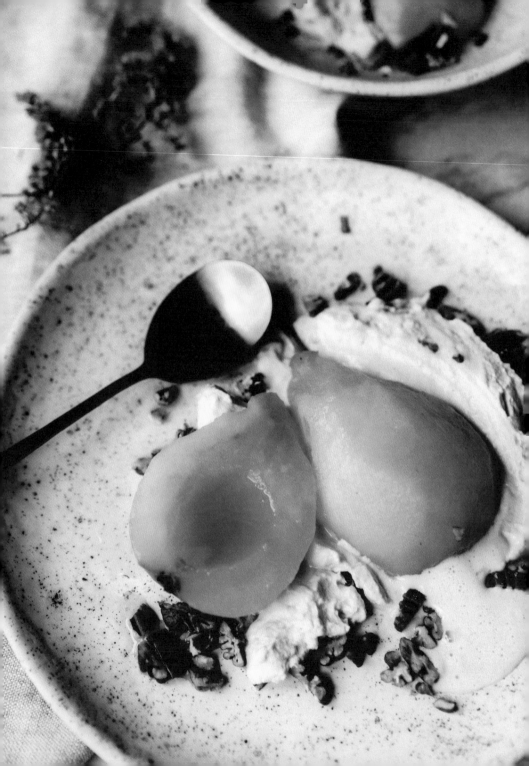

Goldenrod Poached Pears

Makes 4 to 6 servings

Toss the pears with the lemon juice in a large bowl. Set aside. Combine the goldenrod, 2 cups water, wine, honey, cinnamon stick, and ginger in a saucepan over medium heat. Scrape in the seeds from split vanilla bean; add the pod to the saucepan. Stir constantly over medium heat until honey dissolves, about 4 minutes.

Add the pears. Cover and reduce heat to medium-low. Simmer until pears are just tender when pierced with a sharp knife, turning when halfway through cooking, about 15 minutes.

Using a slotted spoon, transfer the pears to a serving bowl. Strain the poaching liquid through a mesh sieve and boil until it's reduced by half, about 20 minutes. Cool the syrup, then pour the syrup over the pears in the serving bowl. Cover and refrigerate until cold, at least 8 hours or up to overnight. Remove the vanilla bean pod. To serve, top with vanilla ice cream or maple whipped cream.

4 small ripe pears, peeled

3 tablespoons fresh lemon juice

½ cup dried goldenrod flowers and leaves, or 1 cup fresh goldenrod

2 cups dry white wine

1 cup honey

1 cinnamon stick, snapped in half

1-inch piece fresh ginger, peeled and chopped

1 vanilla bean, halved lengthwise

Vanilla ice cream or maple whipped cream, for serving

Hawthorn CRATAEGUS CHRYSOCARPA

*F*ound in hedgerows, hawthorn is a prized medicinal tree throughout many cultural traditions as "food for the heart," which has been confirmed by Western medical research. An ally for heartbreak, grief, and a heart that holds too much, hawthorn is a tonic to help us fortify our heart space from a place of protection and nourishment.

With its bright red fruit, hawthorn embodies a strong doctrine of signatures and is the ultimate heart medicine. Used by Indigenous Americans as a "starvation food" when times were lean, it could be eaten fresh or cooked into pies or preserves. In folk medicine, it is considered a cardiotonic for high blood pressure, used over time for the most effectiveness in teas and tinctures. It relaxes and dilates the arteries, increasing the flow of blood to the heart. Used as a circulatory and cardiac herb, it works to normalize blood pressure and enhances memory as it supports general blood flow throughout the body.

CAUTION: Hawthorn is contraindicated for those on pharmaceutical heart and blood pressure medications. Those with heart conditions should seek medical advice before consumption.

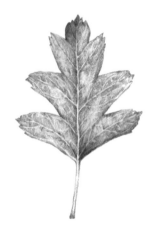

Plant family
Rosaceae

Other names
Thorn apple, cosawa (Ho-Chunk), mayblossom, May tree

Region
Europe, Asia, North America, North Africa

Botanical description
A smaller tree with formidable thorns and a rounded crown. Strong woody, gray trunk; lobed simple green leaves. Clusters of small five-petaled white to light pink flowers bloom in May and ripen into dark red berries in the fall.

Gather
Fleeting flowers bloom in May and the bright red fruit, called haws, ripens in fall.

Herbal actions
Anti-inflammatory, antioxidant, cardio trophorestorative, cardiotonic, hypotensive, nervine, vasodilator

Energetics
Cooling (TCM), warming (Ayurveda), sour

Flower essence
Courage and strength on a spiritual journey

Body systems affinities
Heart chakra, circulatory system

Preparations
Infusion, decoction, syrup, tincture

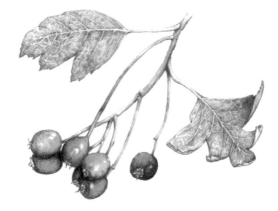

Digging and Processing Roots

We dig the roots in the fall. As we honor our own roots in our ancestors in collective celebration and rituals, we dig the roots of the plants when the energy of the plant dies back into the roots. As flowers and leaves begin to die back, but before a hard frost, is a wonderful time to dig up roots.

Roots can be difficult to lift. It is best to use a long spade, hori hori, or fork to unearth them. Try your best to keep the root intact by gently digging around it. I use digging roots as a meditation to welcome stillness and patience in my body. I ask the roots to release from the earth as I pull them up. If I am too hasty, the roots will snap, but if I approach them with an openness, I can feel them release from the soil.

To clean the root, brush off any mud or soil and wash and scrub the root with a bristled brush. Trim the plant matter from the top. If the root is large, cut it into strips or small pieces. Spread the root out evenly on a drying rack, shelf, or screen and leave in a warm place for 10 days, then turn it and dry for 10 more days—about a full lunar cycle. You will know your roots are dry when they are brittle. Store them in a glass jar with a tight-fitting lid, away from sunlight. Alternatively, roots can be dried in the oven 200 degrees for 4 hours or in a dehydrator to quicken the process.

Mullein VERBASCUM SPP.

*T*all stalks of mullein dot our prairies in midsummer with regality. Mullein leaf is an expectorant and an invaluable herb for congestion and bronchitis, a plant connecting to our throat chakra and inner voice, as the throat chakra includes the ears. Mullein speaks to me of being rooted in ancestral knowledge and listening to the inner voice, a plant to help one who is in avoidance to connect with the truth of a situation, and even their own truths. A biennial plant, growing basal leaves in the first year and yellow flowers during the second year, mullein can be collected and infused in oil to treat ear infections. A compress of mullein leaves can help hemorrhoids.

Mullein is high in vitamin B, magnesium, and vitamin D and can be used in teas and infusions.

CAUTION: Strain the infusion through a muslin cloth; small hairs on mullein leaves can irritate the mouth and throat.

Plant family
Scrophulariaceae

Other names
Velvet leaf

Region
Native to Europe and Asia, naturalized across North America

Botanical description
Upright biennial. First-year basal rosettes have slightly hairy, gray-green lance-shaped leaves; the second year, the tall spikes flower, dotted with bright yellow blooms.

Grow
In well-drained soils, can be grown from seed

Gather
The vibrant leaves in the first-year basal rosette stage or second year before stalks begin to grow. Harvest flowers on second-year stalks.

Herbal actions
Anti-inflammatory, antibiotic, demulcent, astringent, expectorant, nervine, vulnerary, antimicrobial

---

Energetics
Bitter, pungent, cooling, astringent

Flower essence
Staying true to oneself

Preparations
Flowers are edible; also tincture, steams, herbal oil, infusion

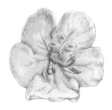

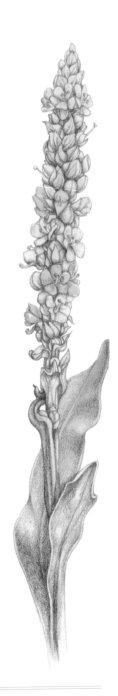

Mushrooms

*U*nlike the immune stimulants elderberry and echinacea, mushrooms are immunomodulators. If you have inflammation or allergies, your immune system is already on high alert. Mushrooms modulate or bring down the response of overactive immune systems or help to increase immune response. They are adaptogenic, meaning they increase nonspecific resilience to stressors and reestablish intrinsic physical, mental, and emotional capacity.

Mushrooms are the fruiting bodies of vast mycelial networks in the ground that act as "highways." Similar to our nervous system that delivers oxygen and hormone messages throughout our bodies, mycelium connects plant roots, sending carbon from mother trees to young trees in times of stress. The fungi networks absorb and store carbon and therefore are an integral part of climate solutions and require our protection as they, too, are under threat from industrial agriculture, pollution, deforestation, and climate change. Harvesting and using the fruiting bodies of mushrooms does not affect the mycelium, and I find working with mushrooms, whether consuming them or visiting them in the forest, brings me feelings of deep peace and connection. I love foraging for mushrooms, but as they are widely cultivated, I buy them fresh at our local farmers' market and food co-op. You can also find a wide array of dried mushrooms that rehydrate when cooked. Before cooking, place them in the midday sun on a patio or a sunny kitchen window to absorb and increase the amount of vitamin D they provide.

CAUTION: Many mushrooms in the wild are poisonous, so please do not harvest or ingest any mushroom you are not 100 percent confident is safe.

LION'S MANE (*HERICIUM ERINACEUS*). Harvest these from summer to late fall; they can be found on decaying hardwood trees like oak, birch, and walnut. Lion's mane is a white, spongy fungus with long tentacles like spines or shaggy teeth hanging down from a central globe. They start to yellow when they are past their prime. Found widely in North America, they have a flavor similar to seafood. Lion's mane is a nootropic mushroom known for boosting memory function and brain health by stimulating the nerve growth factor. It also supports digestive health and the immune system.

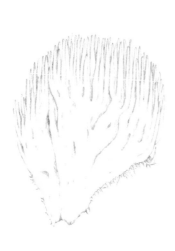

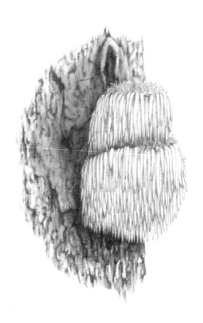

SHIITAKE (*LENTINULA EDODES*). Growing on logs in the forest and easily cultivated in the garden (we have an inoculated shiitake log that sprouts after a good rain), shiitake are tan and brown, umbrella shaped, soft, and spongy. The mushroom cap rolls inward at the edges and has whitish gills on the underside. Valued as a possible anticancer agent, used for centuries in traditional Chinese medicine, and considered an "elixir of life" in Japanese culture, shiitakes are now cultivated worldwide for their many health benefits: They contain iron and vitamin B and are hepatic. They support both the cardiovascular system by regulating cholesterol levels and blood pressure and the immune system by increasing our resistance to bacterial and viral infections. Shiitakes are now widely available in markets and can easily be grown at home from a kit. Use shiitakes in foods, broths, teas, and tinctures.

MAITAKE (*GRIFOLA FRONDOSA*). This mushroom is found at the base of old-growth oaks and maple tree stumps throughout eastern United States, Europe, and Asia in late summer to early autumn. It grows in a cluster of curled and wavy grayish-brown caps. There are no toxic look-alikes for this mushroom; it is a distinct bracket fungus and considered a choice edible. Some can weigh up to one hundred pounds. This is another mushroom I've seen sold at our local market. A very potent medicine for supporting the immune system, it is also anti-inflammatory and anticancer and supports healthy blood sugar, cholesterol, and blood pressure. There is no known toxicity.

Lion's Mane Chowder

I love chowder, but I don't love clams. This recipe is a take on classic clam chowder with lion's mane mushrooms as the stand-in. Lion's mane is a nootropic mushroom with a similar flavor to lobster. I like to blend half the chowder to leave it a little chunky, but feel free to blend it all for a traditional smooth texture.

Makes 6 to 8 servings

In a large Dutch oven, cook the bacon, if using, over medium heat until crisped. Remove the strips and set aside on paper towels to drain; crumble when cool. Using leftover bacon grease or 1 tablespoon of melted butter, sauté the mushrooms, celery, onion, and leek for 5 minutes. Add the butter and garlic, sauté for a minute, and deglaze the pan with the wine.

Add the potatoes, stock, salt, pepper, and thyme sprigs. Bring to a boil, then reduce the heat to medium low to maintain a simmer. Cover and simmer until the potatoes are tender, about 20 minutes. Remove from the heat and take out the sprigs of thyme. With an immersion blender, blend until smooth or leave some chunky if you prefer. Return the chowder to the stovetop.

In a separate bowl, mix together the melted butter and flour into a beurre manié, add it to the chowder, and whisk until activated. Add the milk and continue to cook the chowder over medium heat until it thickens, about 5 minutes, but do not boil. Add cheese at this point, if using. Taste and adjust the seasonings. Garnish with fresh herbs and crumbled bacon.

4 bacon strips (optional)

3 cups chopped lion's mane mushroom

1 cup finely diced celery

1 white onion, finely chopped

1 leek, white part only, well washed and chopped

2 tablespoons butter

4 garlic cloves, finely diced

⅓ cup dry white wine

5 potatoes, chopped

4 cups (32 ounces) chicken or vegetable stock

1 teaspoon sea salt

¼ teaspoon ground white pepper

3 fresh thyme sprigs

1 tablespoon bacon grease or melted butter

⅓ cup all-purpose flour

2 cups whole milk

1 cup shredded organic cheddar cheese (optional)

Chopped fresh dill, tarragon, marjoram, and/or chives, for garnish

Mushroom Galette

Preheat the oven to 400°F.

In a large skillet, melt the butter over medium heat. Add the onions and mushrooms and sauté until they begin to release their juices. Season with sea salt and pepper to taste. Add the thyme and marjoram. Remove from heat and let cool.

On a lightly floured work surface, roll out pastry dough about 12 inches in diameter, leaving a 2 ½-inch-thick border to fold over. Layer the ricotta, mushroom-onion mixture, and sage evenly on the dough. Fold the edges of pastry inward, up and over the filling. If desired, brush the pastry with the egg wash. Bake for 30 to 35 minutes, until crust is golden brown. Serve immediately.

1 tablespoon salted butter

1 small sweet onion, diced

2 cups mushrooms (oyster, cremini, portobello, or shiitake), trimmed and sliced

Sea salt and freshly ground black pepper

1 tablespoon thyme leavess

1 teaspoon dried marjoram

½ cup ricotta (I use a local maple soft sheep's cheese)

3 or 4 fresh sage sprigs, leaves removed and cut into a chiffonade

Piecrust or pastry dough, store-bought or home-made (see page 260)

1 large egg, whisked (optional)

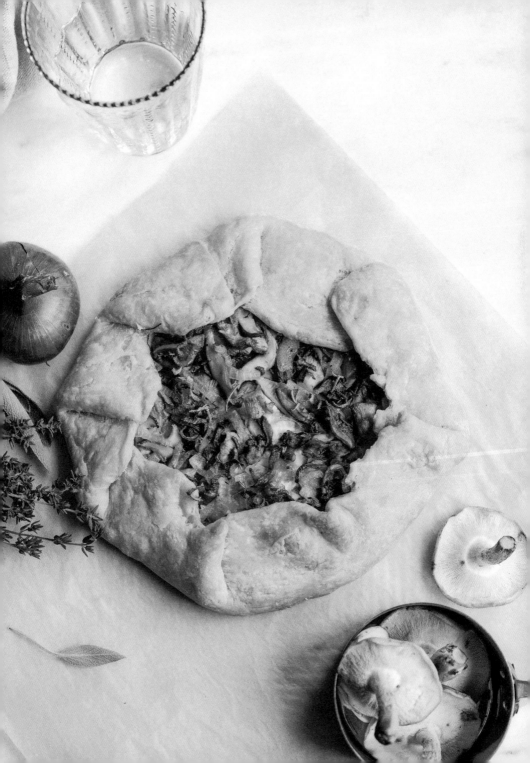

Raspberry Leaf RUBUS IDAEUS

aspberries are a member of the ebullient rose family. With all the sweet fruits it includes, the rose family truly is earth's gift to our heart. Raspberry leaf is a nourishing and tonic herb. Unassuming yet potent, it contains vitamins A, B, C, and E, calcium, iron, phosphorus, potassium, magnesium, selenium, and manganese. A longer infusion that steeps for 4 to 8 hours is a wonderful tonic for low energy levels. One cup of raspberry infusion contains 200 to 250 milligrams of calcium that is easily absorbed by the body.

The Cherokee used raspberry leaf, as well as blackberry leaf or black raspberry leaf, in treating diarrhea through its anti-inflammatory and astringent properties. Its antispasmodic actions ease cramps associated with diarrhea and menstrual pain. It is gentle enough for children's bodies, too. It's also good for mouth ulcers, canker sores, strengthening the gums, sore throats, and balancing menstruation, with its tonifying effects on the womb.

My midwife advised I drink raspberry tea in the last trimester of my pregnancy to help prepare my womb for labor. Raspberry holds us, nourishes us during transformations. Raspberry leaf is a general tonic for the endocrine system, balancing hormones and helping bring irregular cycles back into balance.

CAUTION: For folks with anemia and those with cold and dry energetics, raspberry leaf's high tannin content may interfere with iron absorption.

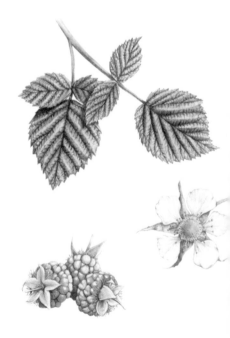

Plant family
Rosaceae

Region
Native to regions of Europe and Asia, black raspberry native to North America

------

Botanical description
Green leaves on the top, silvery gray on the bottom. Pinnate compound with three to five leaflets. Toothed leaves, rounded base with a pointed tip. This rose family flower blooms in spring. Bears red fruits topped with five white petals in the summer and autumn on everbearing thorn-covered canes. When the berry is picked, there is a hollow center.

Grow
Early spring is the best time to plant raspberry in a location with full sun. Soak the roots for an hour before planting. Space raspberry canes 18 to 24 inches apart, leaving plenty of space, as they will spread.

Gather
Begin to harvest raspberry leaves in late spring, summer, and early fall, before the flowers have ripened into berries for the most potent medicine. Try to pick only a few top leaves from each stem, being mindful this is how the plant creates its energy. Leaves can be gathered from both cultivated and wild species.

Herbal actions
Alterative, antispasmodic, astringent, nutritive, tonic

Energetics
Cooling and bitter

Flower essence
Cultivating kindness and compassion for self; releasing old wounds and finding forgiveness for self and others. Brings sweetness to those who are sensitive or take things to heart and lack understanding or are embittered and resentful of others.

Preparations
Tea, infusion, vaginal steam

Tummy Tea

This tea blend is gentle on the stomach relieving indigestion or diarrhea.

Combine the dried herbs and store them in a glass jar. To prepare a cup of tea, mix 2 tablespoons dried herbs and 8 ounces boiling water in a glass jar or vessel. Steep for 20 minutes, strain, and sip.

2 parts dried raspberry leaf

1 part dried chamomile

2 parts dried lemon balm

1 part dried peppermint

Moontime Infusion

This blend is well suited for the menstruating human. I make this blend in the week leading up to my cycle for a nourishing infusion.

Blend the herbs together and store them in an airtight container. To drink, add a heaping tablespoon or 2 to 8 ounces of hot water. Steep for 20 minutes, then strain and add honey.

1 part dried oatstraw

2 parts dried raspberry leaf

2 parts dried nettle

1 part dried rose hips

1 part dried yarrow flowers and leaves

Reishi GANODERMA LUCIDUM

Reishi has been used in traditional Chinese medicine for over 2,000 years and revered in Japanese culture as a bridge between earth and heaven. Called the elixir of life in TCM, reishi is thought to hold the key to immortality. Used to bring the mind and body back into balance, it supports immune response, like allergic reactions, and calms chronic stress and anxiety. Tonifying the heart center, it is now used to lower cholesterol. Reishi, like many mushrooms, are immunomodulating; those properties are best experienced with long-term and daily use. Reishi shines a light, and with its wisdom it lifts our awareness beyond ego, beyond the individual self to our connection with the wider world.

Mushroom polysaccharides are best extracted in hot water. The triterpenes are also extracted in hot water and alcohol. Mushrooms higher in triterpenes are more bitterly flavored, and those high in polysaccharides are more bland tasting. To extract these properties, reishi is best decocted, simmered in water for 20 to 60 minutes before consumption, or use with other herbal ingredients. I love to add reishi decoctions to Elderberry Syrup (page 232) and cook slices of reishi in bone broth for extra immune support.

To make a decoction, bring 2 to 15 grams of chopped reishi mushrooms and 2 liters of water to a boil. Turn down the heat to medium and simmer until the water is reduced by two-thirds.

NOTE
Reishi is not suitable for hemophiliacs or individuals on anticoagulant medications.

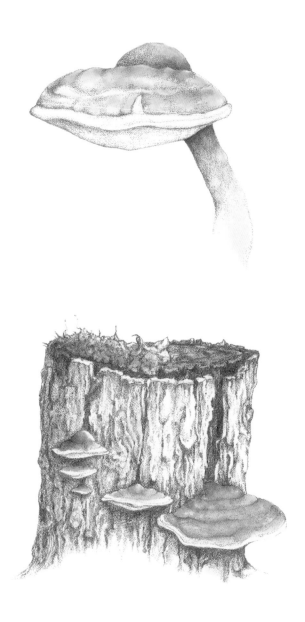

Plant family
Ganodermataceae

- -

Other names
Lingzhi (TCM)

- -

Region
Native to China, Southern Europe, United States

- -

Grow
Lives on dead hardwood trees, often oaks, can be cultivated by inoculating spores into logs.

- -

Botanical description
North American varieties are large and shelflike, while older varieties are smaller with a cap and stalk. A reddish-orange to black fan-shaped semicircular polypore with a cork-like texture, it can be found with or without a lacquered shine. Some varieties have a slender stalk that attaches to the cap from the side. Pores on the underside, not gills. Whitish when fresh and turns brown when aged or bruised.

- -

Gather
Often found on dead oaks. Leave immature mushroom with white stripe around the edge and harvest after it has dropped its spores. Collect after the fruiting body has matured. You can gather it in the wild but be careful not to overharvest. Clean off the dirt, check for insect infestation, dry properly, and store in a cool, dark area.

Herbal actions
Adaptogen, anti-inflammatory, antiviral, cardioprotective, hepatic, hypotensive, immunomodulating, kidney tonic, nervine

- -

Energetics
Bitter, warming, neutral

- -

Flower essence
Supportive in times of transition, revealing hidden connections

- -

Preparations
Tea, infused honey, tincture, syrup, broth, food

Spiced Pumpkin Pie

Truly my kryptonite, I could eat a whole pumpkin pie by myself. I love growing, pureeing, and freezing Long Island cheese pumpkins so I can make pumpkin dishes all winter long. The Long Island cheese pumpkin was the most popular pumpkin to grow for pie before it was replaced with the more commercial sugar pumpkin. This recipe makes two piecrusts; one can be kept in the fridge for two days or in the freezer for two months.

Makes 8 servings

Prepare the piecrust first. Sift together the flour and salt in a large bowl and sprinkle half of the butter on top. Using a pastry blender, mix until the butter is the size of large peas. Add the remaining butter and sprinkle everything with some ice water, a tablespoon or two at a time, blending until the mixture just comes together and the dough pulls away from the sides of the bowl; do not add more water or mix it longer than necessary. Divide the dough in half and wrap each piece separately in plastic wrap, press each into a disk, and place in the refrigerator for at least 30 minutes.

Meanwhile, preheat the oven to 375°F.

Roll out one disk of dough 11 inches round on a lightly floured surface until ⅛ inch thick and transfer it into a 9-inch pie plate, pressing it in evenly and trimming and crimping the edges. Prick the bottom with a fork. Line the pastry with a piece of parchment and pie weights (I use dried black beans). Bake for 20 minutes, remove pie weights and parchment, and let cool.

For the filling, mix all the ingredients together in a large bowl until blended and smooth. Pour the filling into the partially baked piecrust, smoothing the top, and bake for 50 minutes, or until the center is firm. Let the pie cool completely before slicing and serving.

Piecrust

2 cups all-purpose flour, plus more for dusting

½ teaspoon kosher salt

8 tablespoons (1 stick) unsalted butter, chilled and cut into ½ inch pieces

10 tablespoons ice water

Filling

1 (15-ounce) can pumpkin puree, or 2 cups homemade pumpkin puree

½ cup milk (I often use nondairy milk)

3 large eggs

½ cup maple syrup

1 teaspoon ground cinnamon

¾ teaspoon ground ginger

½ teaspoon ground nutmeg

¼ teaspoon ground cardamom

2 tablespoons powdered chaga or reishi mushrooms

¼ teaspoon ground cloves

½ teaspoon kosher salt

1 teaspoon vanilla extract

Rosemary ROSMARINUS OFFICINALE

R osemary is a resilient, drought-resistant plant that can live for years.

Rosemary was originally cultivated on the shores of the Mediterranean. The Latin name, *Rosmarinus*, is derived from the words *ros*, meaning "dew," and *marinus*, which means "sea," as rosemary can survive on the spray of the sea air. It's a hardy plant that I consider one of my first plant allies.

A tonic and stimulating herb, bringing vitality to life and known for its culinary uses, it is antibacterial and antifungal. Rosemary is used for cleansing, release, remembrance, memory, and psychic, spiritual, and physical purification.

A warming herb that improves circulation and digestion and clears stagnation in the mind and body, massaging the body with rosemary oil will increase circulation, relieve aches and pains, and warm the limbs. If you are feeling lethargic, bored, or uninspired, a single inhale can awaken your senses. Rosemary can help lift one from depression and enhance the mind. Its bitter taste aids in digestion, stimulates the liver, and using it in cooking helps balance meals.

Rosemary's flower essence supports one who is exhausted or weary or feeling burdened by the weight of the world. It builds resilience for living and provides emotional balance and a calming energy.

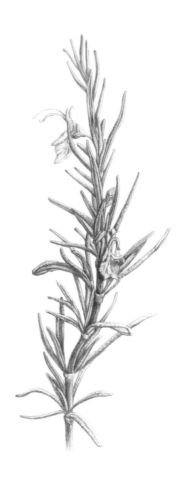

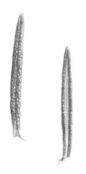 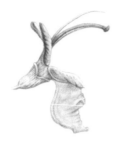 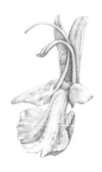

Plant family
Lamiaceae

Other names
Compass weed,
dew of the sea

Region
Native to the Mediterranean,
naturalized in Europe, Asia,
and America

Botanical description
Aromatic, shrubby, evergreen
perennial with narrow, dark
green leaves about 1 inch
long, with pine-like leaflets
and blue mouth-shaped
flowers

Grow
Start seeds indoors 8 to
10 weeks before the last frost
or outdoors any time after
the last frost. This tender
perennial prefers full sun and
soil with not too much acidity.
Here in the Midwest in the
fall, I dig my rosemary and
pot it to overwinter it. I keep
it alive in the winter months
by misting the plant with
water. The plant takes in
water from its aerial parts and
prefers dry soil. I water it
every other week and mist its
leaves regularly.

Parts used
Leaves

Gather
Harvest leaves in the spring
through the fall. Where I
grew up in California,
rosemary could be harvested
and bloomed into the winter
months.

Herbal actions
Antidepressant, anti-
inflammatory, antioxidant,
astringent, carminative,
emmenagogue, nervine,
stimulant

Energetics
Bitter and warming

Flower essence
Warming the spirit and
clearing away the fog;
grounding in your essence
and connecting to your
lineage

Preparations
Culinary uses are endless!
Also tea, infusion, and infused
vinegar

Roasted Cranberry and Rosemary Shrub

I love adding this tart syrup to champagne during the holidays. The discarded cranberries are yummy, too.

2 cups fresh cranberries

1 cup honey

4 fresh rosemary sprigs, leaves removed and chopped

1 cup apple cider vinegar

Makes about 10 servings

Preheat the oven to 375°F. Line a baking sheet with parchment paper and spread the cranberries out on it. Roast for 20 minutes, or until the cranberries have popped and released some juices. Remove the baking sheet from the oven and place the cranberries in a bowl. Pour the honey and chopped rosemary over the cranberries and mix well. Cover the bowl with a kitchen towel and let it sit overnight so the cranberries release their juices.

Pour the cranberry mixture into a glass jar and add the cider vinegar. Cover with a plastic lid, shake, and refrigerate overnight, then strain the mixture through a fine-mesh sieve into a bottle or jar, pressing out as much juice as possible, and store in the refrigerator for up to 2 weeks. To use the shrub, add 3 tablespoons to 8 ounces sparkling water. You can also add a splash of something stronger if you prefer.

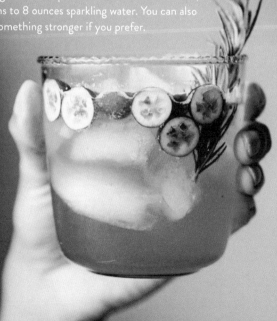

Sage SALVIA OFFICINALIS

A prized culinary and medicinal herb throughout the centuries, sages grow in grasslands, prairies, and even desert climates. There are more than 900 species of sage, many of which play important roles in sacred ceremonies and spiritual rituals. Cultivated varieties of sage are grown in gardens. Sage moves digestive and respiratory stagnation and can help move stuck emotions, clearing the mind and heart. Sage is used for sore throats, can support us in using our voices, and acts as a balancing herb—if you are warm, it will have a cooling effect in the body; if you are cool, it will promote circulation. It works well to dry up mucous membranes and heaviness due to damp head colds. Sage honey in tea is perfect for soothing sore throats.

Sage's constituents can be easily extracted. Good for common colds as well as for preparing sacred spaces, sage is burned across cultures to cleanse and purify. Sage smoke helps us communicate by carrying our messages and prayers.

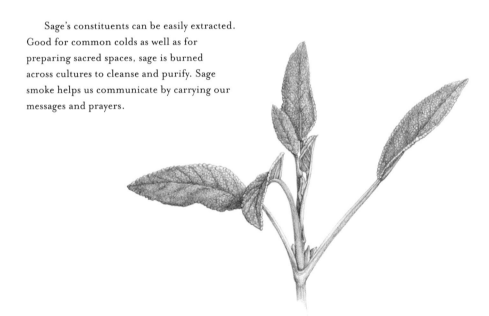

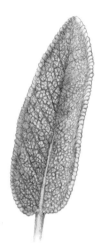

Plant family
Lamiaceae

Region
The common garden and culinary sage used today is native to Eurasia, spread to Europe, and is now cultivated worldwide. There are more than 900 species of sage growing in grasslands with well-drained soils.

Botanical description
Sage has square stems, a common feature of the Lamiaceae family, and alternating, opposite, toothed ovate leaves that are furry, light green.

Grow
Start seeds indoors 6 to 10 weeks or outdoors 1 to 2 weeks before the last frost. This easy-to-grow perennial prefers well-drained soil and full to partial sunlight.

Gather
Leaves throughout the summer and fall; when cut they grow back quickly. Bundle the leaves and dry them upside down.

Herbal actions
Antibiotic, antifungal, anti-inflammatory, antimicrobial, antioxidant, antiseptic, bitter, carminative, digestive, diuretic, expectorant, nervine

Energetics
Pungent, aromatic, bitter, drying

Flower essence
To open intuition and to access wisdom deep within the body and from life experiences; clear your channels; drawing wisdom from experience

Preparations
Tea, tincture, infused honey, infused oil, steam, vinegar, in cooking

Herbal Macaroni and Cheese

This recipe is my herbal adaptation of my mom's family's favorite baked macaroni and cheese, which she makes for our holiday gatherings. Macaroni and cheese has its historical roots in African American cuisine, and this recipe celebrates the fact that comfort food can be herbal, too.

Makes 8 servings

Preheat the oven to 350°F. Bring a large pot of water to a boil and add salt to taste and the elbow macaroni. Cook until al dente, according to package instructions, stirring occasionally. Drain the pasta and set aside.

Melt 1 tablespoon of the butter in a large saucepan over medium heat. Add ¼ cup of the chopped sage and the garlic. Sauté for about 1 minute. Add the wine and simmer until it is reduced by half, 2 to 3 minutes.

Add the milk and continue to cook until it returns to a light simmer. Take the skillet off the heat, pour the contents into a blender and blend until smooth, then pour it back into the skillet. Add the remaining 3 tablespoons butter, the cheddar cheese, 1 cup of the Gouda, the nutmeg, paprika, and pepper and stir until the sauce has thickened.

Stir in the al dente macaroni and pour everything into a 9 × 13-inch baking dish. Make sure there is enough milk and add more if needed because the pasta will soak it up quickly and make the dish dry. Top with the remaining 2 cups Gouda, sprinkle with panko and sage and thyme. Bake for 30 minutes, or until the panko is browned and the sauce is bubbling.

Kosher salt

1 (1-pound) box elbow macaroni

4 tablespoons (½ stick) butter

¼ cup finely chopped fresh sage

1 garlic clove, finely minced

½ cup dry white wine

1¼ cups whole milk, plus more if needed

2 cups shredded sharp white cheddar cheese

3 cups shredded Gouda cheese

⅛ teaspoon ground nutmeg

⅛ teaspoon paprika

Freshly ground black pepper

½ cup panko breadcrumbs, for topping

¼ cup mixed finely chopped mixed fresh sage and thyme, for topping

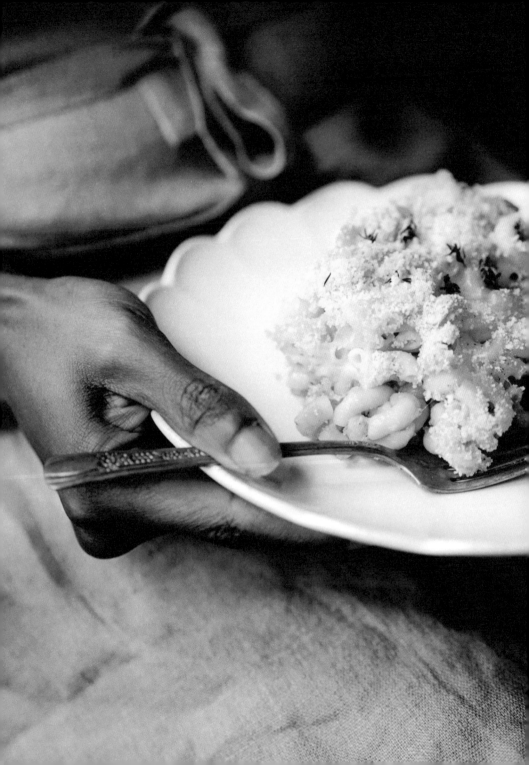

Sumac RHUS SPP

S umac grows in colonies along the roadsides, on prairies, and at the fields' edges here in the Midwest. All edible sumacs have reddish-purple fruits called drupes. Harvest when they are bright red for the lemony flavor; the flavor fades as the drupes darken. Sumac was used in South African materia medica for kidney problems

Well known and loved in Middle Eastern cuisine and used extensively in Indigenous ethnobotany as a spice, often in rubs for meats and fish, sumac has a citrus flavor and a cooling effect. It's a wonderful ingredient for sumac lemonade, offering a cooling respite, clearing feelings of heaviness, and bringing clarity.

Due to its polyphenols, flavonoids, and free-radical-scavenging effects, "modern research highlights sumac as a promising antioxidant for chronic diseases such as atherosclerosis and diabetes."

Sumac can be used to cool fevers and soothe inflamed stomach and urinary tract tissues.

CAUTION: Poison sumac has white berries, not red. All edible sumac have red fruits.

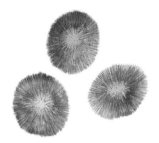

Plant family
Anacardiaceae

- - - - - - - - - - - - - - - - - - - -

Other names
Staghorn sumac, lemonade berry, scarlet sumac

- - - - - - - - - - - - - - - - - - - -

Region
Grows in temperate regions worldwide

- - - - - - - - - - - - - - - - - - - -

Botanical description
A deciduous shrub that grows in groupings along roadside, at the prairie's edge, and in areas with disturbed soils. Its light brown bark turns gray as it ages. Sumac has cone-like burgundy-red fruits, or

drupes. Leaves are alternate, large and long, serrated and lanceolate, a glossy green that turns red in autumn.

- - - - - - - - - - - - - - - - - - - -

Gather
USDA Hardiness Zones 5 to 8. Sumac berries are ready for picking from late summer to early fall. If you've harvested a bunch of these beautiful red berries, you can dry and grind them up to use as a lemony-earthy flavored spice, or use them immediately to make a tangy and refreshing beverage.

Herbal actions
Antiviral, anti-inflammatory, antioxidant, antimicrobial.

- - - - - - - - - - - - - - - - - - - -

Energetics
Cool, dry, sour, astringent

- - - - - - - - - - - - - - - - - - - -

Flower essence
The courage to step out into the world

- - - - - - - - - - - - - - - - - - - -

Body systems affinities
Kidney, bladder, liver, lungs

- - - - - - - - - - - - - - - - - - - -

Preparations
Seasoning, tea

Sumac and Sage Salt

Herbal salts are a good way to incorporate nutrition and flavor into your daily meals. I love the citrus notes of sumac and the earthy flavors of sage.

Mix all the ingredients together and store them in an airtight jar. Sprinkle on meats and vegetables when roasting.

2 tablespoons ground sumac

1 tablespoon ground sage

1 teaspoon kosher salt flakes

1 teaspoon garlic powder (optional)

Roasted Squash with Sumac Seasoning

Makes 4 servings

Preheat the oven to 400°F. Cut the squash in half, scoop out and discard the seeds and fibrous interior, and slice it thinly. Arrange the squash in a single layer on a baking sheet. Top the squash with the sliced butter and scatter on the sage leaves. Season to taste with the sumac-sage salt and pepper.

Roast for 40 minutes, until soft and golden. Sprinkle with nettle seasoning, if using, and serve.

2 pounds squash

2 tablespoons salted butter, sliced

5 small fresh sage leaves

Sumac and Sage Salt (above)

Freshly ground black pepper

Nettle Seasoning (page 125; optional)

Sumac Lemonade

Makes 2 servings

Place the rinsed sumac berries and 2 cups cool water in a large jar. One large cluster of sumac will flavor a minimum of 2 cups water; the more sumac you use, the quicker and more flavorful the lemonade will be.

Soak the sumac in water for at least a few hours. Strain through cheesecloth, coffee filter, or similar fine-mesh fabric into a jar or pitcher; discard the solids. Once it's strained, sweeten to taste with honey or maple syrup. Serve chilled or over ice and enjoy.

1 cluster (about 1 cup) fresh sumac berries (drupes), rinsed to remove debris

Honey or maple syrup, to taste

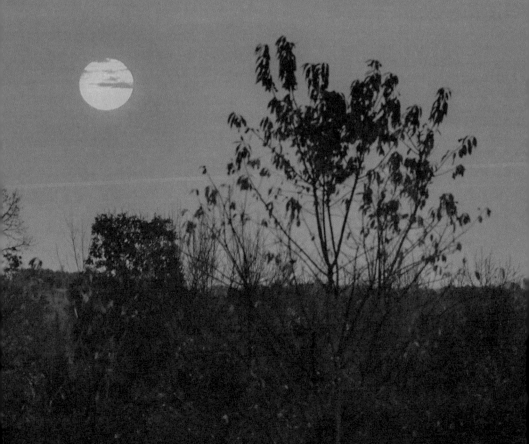

Thyme THYMUS VULGARIS

*T*hyme is an aromatic, savory, warming herb that supports the healthy functioning of our lungs. It is a drying expectorant, antispasmodic and antimicrobial. Its primary biological constituent, thymol, is an expectorant for the lungs, and its anti-inflammatory effects aid in relieving chest congestion, bronchitis, coughs, and indigestion.

According to several studies done by Dr. Paul Lee, a professor at the University of California Santa Cruz, thyme has a strengthening effect on the thymus gland, which boosts immune function. Thyme can also be used externally as a disinfectant. I trim my thyme plant back a couple times in the summer season, hanging it to dry and use in cooking. It's best harvested before it flowers, but I love using the edible flowers in salad as well.

In Ayurvedic medicine, thyme is considered an antiseptic, astringent, and expectorant. It reduces vata (air) and kapha (earth). An Ayurvedic remedy for treating coughs uses a drop or two of thyme essential oil in a facial steam.

You can make thyme cough syrup by combining 1 ounce of fresh thyme sprigs and 3 cups of water, simmering about 15 minutes. Let the decoction sit, then strain through cheesecloth into a pint-size jar. Stir in ½ cup of raw honey until dissolved, and store the syrup in the refrigerator for up to 6 weeks. Take 1 teaspoon every few hours for respiratory ailments.

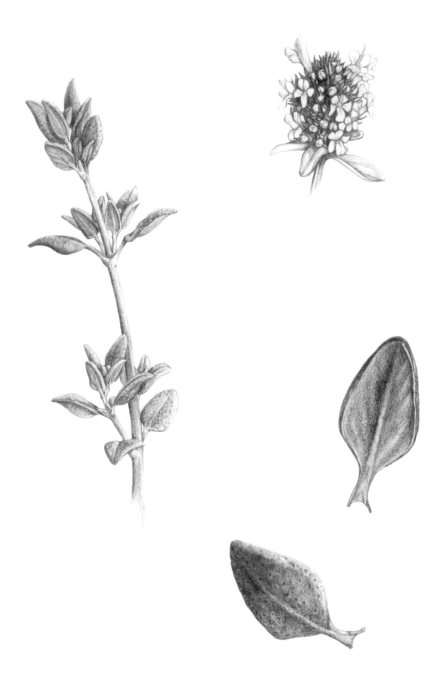

Plant family
Lamiaceae

Other names
Creeping thyme, wild thyme

Region
Native to Europe and Asia; widely cultivated and a favorite in cottage gardens

Botanical description
A small, low-growing shrub akin to ground cover. Woody base and simple, ovate, grayish-green opposite leaves ½ inch long. Characteristics of mint family flowers, the tiniest of white to purple whorled flowers cluster together.

Grow
Start seeds indoors 6 to 10 weeks or outside 2 to 3 weeks before last frost. This perennial prefers fertile, dry soil and grows in partial to full sun. Thyme is drought and frost resistant.

Gather
Cut vibrant tops at any point from summer to fall. I will often do my last harvest close to the first frost of autumn.

Herbal actions
Anti-inflammatory, antioxidant, antimicrobial, antiparasitic, antispasmodic, astringent, carminative, diaphoretic, expectorant

Energetics
Warming and drying

Flower essence
Release struggle in preparation for action

Body systems affinities
Respiratory, immune, digestive

Preparations
As a culinary herb, used as seasoning for poultry, soups, and sauces; infused vinegar, infused honey

Épis

Used in everything from seasonal soups to meats, épis is a staple in every Haitian kitchen. The smell reminds me of my grandmother's kitchen. I love eating this scrambled into eggs. Sautéed épis is also a delish base for beans, soups, and stews.

Makes 1 quart

In the bowl of a food processor fitted with an S blade, combine the parsley, bell peppers, onion, thyme, scallions, garlic, cloves, celery (if using), bouillon (if using), and Scotch bonnet (if using).

Pulse (not puree) to chop the vegetables into smaller pieces. Slowly pour in the olive oil and vinegar. Continue to pulse until the mixture is blended but with a chunky texture resembling pesto. Store the épis in a large glass jar in the refrigerator or freeze it in ice cube trays. The épis will keep for 2 weeks in the refrigerator and 1 month in the freezer.

1 cup chopped parsley

2 bell peppers, sliced

1 small onion, chopped

10 fresh thyme sprigs

3 scallions, sliced

6 garlic cloves

3 whole cloves

1 or 2 celery stalks (optional)

1 bouillon cube, or 2 tablespoons stock base paste (optional)

¼ to ½ Scotch bonnet chile pepper (optional)

⅓ cup olive oil

3 tablespoon apple cider vinegar, lime juice, or a mix of both

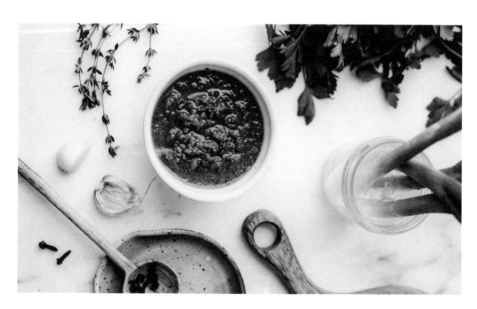

Winter

*The Season
of the North*

⋮

New Moon

⋮

Yin

⋮

*Dreaming,
Contemplation,
Inner Work*

Seasonal Wisdom

Plunged into darkness, we gather the pieces of ourselves and release old skins to find grains of truth to plant when spring returns.

Winter solstice
Around December 21

Astrology of winter
Capricorn (cardinal earth), Aquarius (fixed air), Pisces (mutable water)

Energetics of winter
Cold becoming wet

Element
Air

Chakra
Third eye and crown

In December, we welcome the Cold Moon or Long Night Moon as we approach the winter solstice and the longest night of the year. Rosehips have been sweetened with a first frost; they are ready to be plucked from their thorny abode.

Unlike winters of our ancestors' past, modern Decembers are filled with expectation and mass consumption. How can we cultivate a less-hurried pace of life? Shift our focus on gathering over consumption? What can you make rather than what can you buy? Building traditions, cultivating community, and rituals around connecting with our inner light and nourishing ourselves. Making gifts of collected seeds and homemade jams, tea blends grown in our gardens and crafted with heart, hand-rolled beeswax candles and forced bulbs. Hand-sewn lavender eye pillows, sourdough starters, and herbal bundles to burn.

Winter is a time to dream, to connect to old memories, to journey inward. Soils rest and souls lie fallow. We rest our bodies to replenish our souls. It is a time for reflection. I step outside, enlivened by the frigid morning air, to sip coffee as the sun begins to rise in the east and the moon sets in the west behind the trees.

Focus on cultivating your inner light, connecting, and creating cozy moments. Root into stillness and reflect on the season's past. We begin to dream and plan for the season ahead. It is a season of welcoming little deaths and calling ourselves back home. This is truly a season of deep listening and resonance that can be overshadowed by too much consumption and commercialization. For me, winter becomes a season of cultivating personal rituals and family traditions to divest and practice setting healthy boundaries. It is an opportunity to deeply listen to the needs of myself and my family. Eat by candlelight and learn to tap into other senses.

Winter is the season of tea. I wrap my cold hands around warm mugs filled with nourishing beverages while the skies are gray and the night sets in earlier. Ward off winter blues with warming foods and herbal preparations like St. John's wort and lemon balm. This time is spent deep in our roots and keeping warm near the hearths of our home. Take winter walks in the cold, brisk fresh air and go owling at night.

In February, a Hunger Moon rises in the sky. Although it is still a time for reflection and stillness, a sense of anticipation arises within us. For our ancestors, this is when food stores could become scarce. Tend closely to yourself and your mental health. A sense of restlessness sets in as I begin to dream of garden plans and planting seeds. For encouragement, bring life into the home, branches of flowering trees or bulbs tucked in to force their blooms. Start microgreens of arugula and broccoli on the windowsill for some nutrients as the sun's energy slowly begins to grow in the sky again.

As the season of winter shifts into spring, it is still a time to rest and digest the year gone by and to hold fast to our dreams for the season ahead.

Chaga INONOTUS OBLIQUUS

Chaga is a parasitic fungus that grows on birch trees and takes decades to reach maturity. If a birch tree is infected with different medicinal mushrooms, chaga will not be found there.

I have an abiding connection with chaga. To me, chaga feels like a deep embrace. It supports immune function without overstimulating the immune system and soothes the digestive tract. It has an affinity for the lungs and heart and is cardioprotective. Chaga imparts a deep sense of ease and grounding, but I don't use it as often as I would like due to issues with sustainability and overharvesting. In honoring the sacred nature of this plant and its life cycle, I abstain from frequent use.

We must be mindful of how we extract, consume, and use all things, especially plants. I try not to use chaga powder, instead making a decoction with chunks of locally and sustainably harvested chaga. I use three or four chunks in a big slow cooker full of water to make tea, and I can reuse the chunks a couple times. I sweeten it with maple syrup, a dash of cinnamon, and warm oat milk.

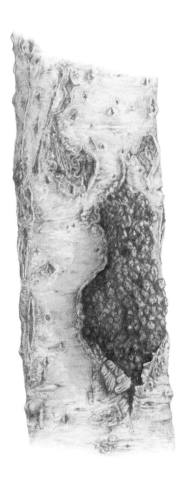

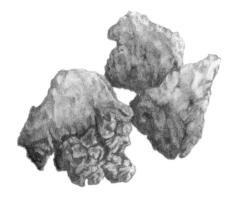

Plant family
Hymenochaetaceae

Other names
Bai hua rong, tinder conk,
black mass

Region
Grows on birch in Europe,
Russia, Asia, and North
America

Botanical description
Black, charred appearance on
the outside; soft, spongelike
orange or gold core

Gather
Chaga faces hard pressure
from wildcrafting as it is a
slow-growing fungus, choose
other herbs or fungi, if
they're available. It takes
decades for chaga to reach
maturity, which, similar to
wild ramps, brings up
conversations about
sustainable and ethical
harvesting and usage.

Herbal actions
Adaptogen, anticarcinogenic,
antitumor, antiviral, immune
tonic, immunomodulating

Energetics
Neutral

Preparations
Decoction, broth, tea

Pine PINUS SPP.

An evergreen tree, a symbol of life through cold, hard winters, pine trees are primarily found in the Northern Hemisphere. With over 250 species globally, they are the most abundant member of the conifer family. Pine is a living embodiment of rootedness and deep time, a manifestation of sovereignty among a whole. Pine trees keep their needles for two years; as older needles fall, new ones grow in. They are well adapted to cold climates and poor soils.

Pines evolved some 90 million years ago, an elder of the forest, the great tree of peace to the Haudenosaunee Nations. The most commonly used pine in Western herbalism is the eastern white pine, yet all pines can be used. Pine is used in both Native American and African American herbal traditions as nutritive food and healing medicine for coughs, colds, viral infections, chest congestions, and respiratory ailments, especially in the winter months. Pine wisdom is a reminder that even in the darkest months, there is hope. Pine trees are intertwined with the history of colonization and the lumber industry in the United States, as logged pine provided shelter and fueled expansion and settler colonialism, so much so that eastern pine old-growth forests are nonexistent.

Pine tops can be harvested in the spring, and fresh needles, along with the sap, seeds (commonly known as pine nuts), and resin can be used. Its clusters of two to five soft needles are wrapped in a paperlike sheath at the base. When a tree is wounded, pine resin flows to the surface to seal the wound from organisms, a doctrine of signatures indicating its topical antibacterial use for skin, wounds, and infections as well as for muscle aches and pains. Pine needles are an excellent source of vitamin C, which aids the immune system. Pine can be used for intestinal worms, skin conditions, and fungal infections.

I connect with the pine before I harvest, giving thanks, my respect, honor, and prayers, and ask for permission from the plant. The fresh needles are more tender and a lighter color when steamed. White pine is wonderful for digestion and a mild expectorant for wet coughs.

I invite you to enter into relationship with a conifer tree beyond hosting it in your house for the holidays, as their wisdom and healing powers are immense.

CAUTION: All pine species are safe. The yew tree resembles pine but is toxic; it has smaller, flat needles and little red berries.

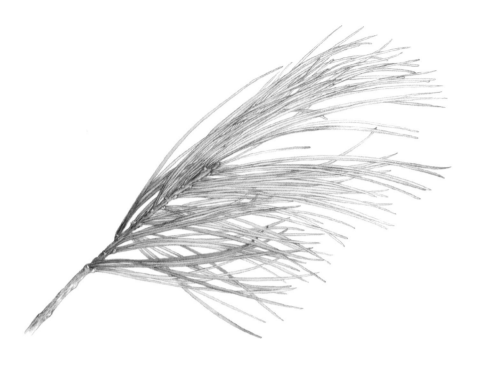
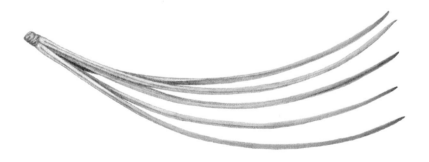

Plant family
Pinaceae

Other names
Zhingwaak in Ojibwe

Region
USDA Hardiness Zones 4 to 9; in temperate and boreal forests throughout North America, China, Southeast Asia, Russia, and Europe

---

Botanical description
Long, narrow needles up to 11 inches in length. Different species of pine have different groupings of needles. Eastern white pine needles are grouped in fives in a paperlike sheath at the base, where they connect and attach to the branch.

Gather
Pine needles year-round, particularly in spring and winter; resin, pollen, seeds

---

Herbal actions
Anti-inflammatory, antimicrobial, antispasmodic, antiseptic, antiviral, circulatory stimulant, expectorant, immune support

Energetics
Pungent, stimulating, warming

Flower essence
For those who blame themselves

Preparations
Tea, syrup, infused oil, steam bath, bath salts, salve, baked goods

Pine Needle Tea

The evergreen needles of pine are a balm on gray days. We enjoy this tea around bonfires on chilly winter days. Pine's citrus flavor is uplifting and nourishing in the doldrums of winter.

2 to 4 tablespoons washed and chopped fresh white pine needles (see Note)

4 slices fresh ginger

1 teaspoon dried orange peel, or a fresh lemon slice

½ cinnamon stick

Honey or maple syrup

Makes 2 cups

In a large kettle, boil a little more than 2 cups of water.

Combine the pine needles, ginger, orange peel, and cinnamon stick in a saucepan or a pot, cover with boiling water and boil on the stovetop for 3 minutes, then remove from the heat. Cover and steep for 15 to 20 minutes, then pour the mixture through a fine-mesh strainer; compost the spent herbs. Pour into two mugs. Infuse your intention for the tea and for your day, placing a stone near the tea to affirm your intention.

Add a dollop of honey or maple syrup and enjoy the tea in a peaceful place, connecting with the essence of the plant and noticing its effects on your mind, body, and spirit.

NOTE
The more finely chopped the pine needles, the more flavor is released.

Fever Tea

An herbal combination shared with me by a friend, this tea is truly a life saver. This cooling and carminative combination helps with sickness and fevers.

1 part dried yarrow

1 part dried elderflowers

1 part dried mint

Cinnamon sticks, to harmonize flavor (optional)

In a jar, mix the herbs together and store. To soothe a fever, add a spoonful to 8 ounces boiling water and let steep for 5 to 10 minutes. Strain, then serve with a teaspoon of honey.

Pine Needle Cough Syrup

Pine needle syrup is a favorite in our home during the winter months. Magnolia, Griffin, and I hike on our path to one of our favorite spots with a stand of pine trees. The kids sit under the pines while I harvest needles from the tree. We make this pine needle cough syrup for winter colds and immune support—and because it tastes delicious.

1 cup washed and chopped fresh pine needles

1 cup honey

Makes 2 cups

Place the chopped pine needles in a saucepan and cover with 2 cups water. Bring to a simmer over medium heat, cover, and cook for 20 to 30 minutes. Remove from the heat, let cool slightly, and strain through a fine-mesh sieve into a jar or airtight container. Add the honey and stir until thoroughly combined. Store in the refrigerator for up to 2 months.

Nourishing Winter Bath

Makes about 2 cups or 1 pint jar

In a blender, combine the oats, calendula, and dried lavender and blend to a fine powder. Pour this into a medium bowl and stir in the remaining ingredients. Store the mixture in a pint glass jar. When ready for a restorative bath, add ½ cup to your tub, using a mesh strainer to save finicky plumbing. Soak and enjoy.

½ cup rolled oats

¼ cup dried calendula

⅛ cup dried lavender buds

1 cup Epsom salts

½ cup French green clay

1 teaspoon almond oil

5 drops lavender essential oil

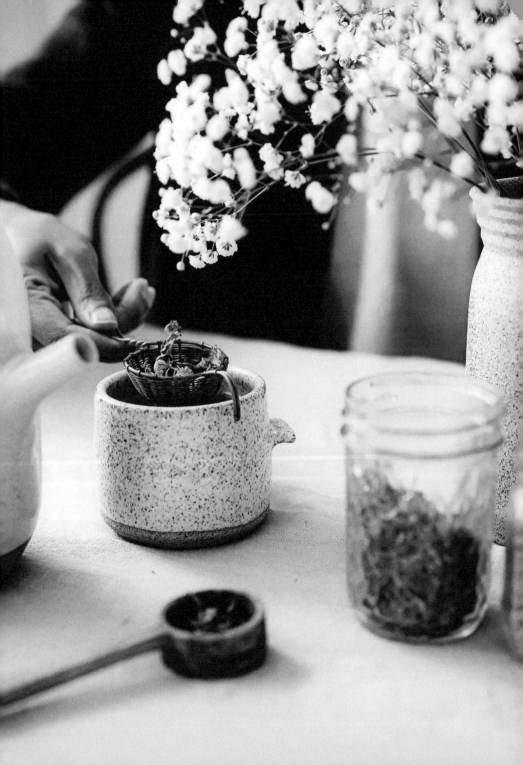

Pine Spritz Cookies

These cookies are a delightful addition to our winter traditions.
Harvest fresh and bright white pine needles. If you do not have
access to pine, rosemary is a fine alternative.

Makes 24 cookies

Preheat the oven to 325°F. In a large mixing bowl, cream together the butter, cream cheese, and sugar with an electric mixer until light and fluffy, about 5 minutes. Add the egg yolk, vanilla, orange zest, and pine needles. Beat until just combined. Add the flour and salt and stir just until all the ingredients are combined.

Follow the manufacturer's instructions for using the cookie press and press out cookies onto cold, unlined, ungreased baking sheets, about 1 inch apart from each other (they shouldn't spread too much). Once the cookies are on the baking sheets, you can add sprinkles or decorate with sugar.

Bake for 12 to 15 minutes. They will be light in color on top and just a little golden underneath. Be careful not to overcook. Remove with a spatula and let cool on a wire rack. Store in an airtight container.

1 cup (2 sticks) unsalted butter, at room temperature

1 (8-ounce) package full-fat cream cheese, at room temperature

1 cup sugar

1 egg yolk

1 teaspoon vanilla extract

Zest of 1 orange

¼ cup powdered pine needles

2½ cups all-purpose flour

¼ teaspoon salt

Sprinkle or sugar, for decoration

Electrolyte Drink

One winter, everyone in our house went down with a horrible stomach flu—except me. Round after round, waking up to sickness, it lasted for almost a month. I made this recipe quite a few times in that stretch instead of buying sugary electrolyte drinks from the market. This is simple, can be made in the middle of the night with items in the pantry, and will help those sick stay hydrated.

32 ounces soothing herbal tea, like chamomile, or water

1 teaspoon honey or maple syrup

½ teaspoon kosher sea salt

Makes 4 servings

Combine all the ingredients in a quart-size glass jar, shake well, and refrigerate. Give just a small amount at a time to help rehydrate during a stomach flu or other digestive problems.

Herbal Electuary

An electuary is a medicinal preparation made with honey. Mix this potent and shelf-stable blend of powdered herbs and spices in honey into your morning coffee, black tea, or straight into water for an instant beverage. My herbal suggestions include rose, sage, cinnamon, turmeric, and ginger—all either ground or powdered,

2 to 3 tablespoons ground herbs of your choice

Organic honey

Place the herbs in a bowl. Slowly pour in honey, stirring just enough so a paste forms. When it is thick and fully incorporated, it's done. Store the electuary in a clean, sterilized half-pint jar in the refrigerator for up to 12 months.

Forcing Spring Bulbs

In the autumn, when I dig trenches under the full Harvest Moon and plant my spring bulbs, I tuck a few away to force indoors, tricking them into blooming out of season. Paperwhites are the most common forced bulb, but I've saved my daffodil varieties, too. Paperwhites belong to the Amaryllis family, which you may be familiar with as it includes some of the first blooms in the spring: the daffodil, the jonquil, and the paperwhite, symbolizing hope in the darkness of winter.

Because paperwhites do not require a cooling period like their kin, they are easiest to force indoors, although I do save daffodil bulbs from our autumn planting, cool them in the refrigerator for a period, and force-bloom them in January. Paperwhites emerge as they are planted, with flowers appearing in 3 to 4 weeks.

Take a vessel of your choosing, such as a jar, low bowl, or pot, and fill it with about 2 inches of washed gravel or stones; this is the minimum amount of space the root system will need. Nestle the paperwhite bulbs into the jar pointed end up; they can grow closely together in widemouthed jars. Add water until it reaches just the base of the bulbs, the bulbs will spread their roots down and through the rocks. Be cautious: bulbs sitting in soggy conditions can rot.

Set the container in indirect light. Check the bulbs frequently, as growing bulbs can dry out within a day or two, and water them only when dry. Water with a mixture of five parts water to one part vodka when the leaves and flower spikes appears. This will help the paperwhite grow straight and compact, not topple over. Then place them in a sunny windowsill and watch them grow.

These make a great gift, bringing a spark of hope on dreary winter days.

Warming Salve

WITH CALENDULA OIL, ROSEMARY OIL, GINGER, AND CAYENNE

I love this salve in the depths of winter when my energy is lower and my body is stagnant. Rosemary is a circulatory herb, and the ginger, calendula, and cayenne are warming. This is perfect to rub on achy muscles.

1 cup carrier oil of choice

1 tablespoon dried rosemary leaves

1 tablespoon dried calendula flowers

1 tablespoon ground cayenne pepper

1 tablespoon ground ginger

¼ cup beeswax

Essential oil (optional)

Makes 5 (2-ounce) tins

Fill a saucepan a quarter of the way with water and bring it to a boil. Place your carrier oil and herbs into a second, smaller saucepan, a glass bowl that fits inside your saucepan, or a double boiler. Use a spoon to mix the herbs and oil together. Heat the smaller saucepan over simmering water for 30 to 60 minutes, making sure no water splashes in. When the infusion is complete, strain the oil into a bowl through a muslin-lined mesh strainer, making sure to press on the solids and squeeze out as much oil as possible. Strain again to remove any sediment and compost.

In a clean saucepan or bowl set over simmering water, combine the infused oil and beeswax, stirring until the beeswax is melted. Add a few drops of essential oil, if using, and then pour the salve into 1-ounce jars or tins to cool. Once cooled, cover and label the jars or tins. Apply small amounts to areas of chronic pain and aching joints, taking care not to use it around the eyes or on your face. Always wash your hands after application.

Herbal Hot Chocolate

Hot chocolate is a favorite treat during winter. After ice skating or a winter woodland walk, the children always ask for a fire in the hearth and a mug of hot chocolate. Using chocolate in this recipe makes it decadent and smooth. I love infusing winter beverages with herbal allies to support the mood. I often use holy basil for the dried herbs in this recipe, but lavender, peppermint, or anise hyssop would also be nice.

3 cups milk
(I prefer oat milk)

2 tablespoons dried herbs

3 ounces chocolate, chopped
(I use Lily's sugar-free milk chocolate or dark chocolate)

Whipped cream and/or marshmallows, for serving (optional)

Makes 2 servings

In a saucepan, gently heat your milk over low heat, add the dried herbs, and let the milk steam. Do not bring to a boil or scald. Remove from the heat and cover the pan, letting the herbs infuse for 10 minutes. Strain the milk through a cheesecloth-lined sieve. Return the infused milk to the pot over low heat and whisk in the chopped chocolate until melted, smooth, and incorporated. Remove from the heat and pour into mugs. Top with marshmallows and whipped cream, if you desire.

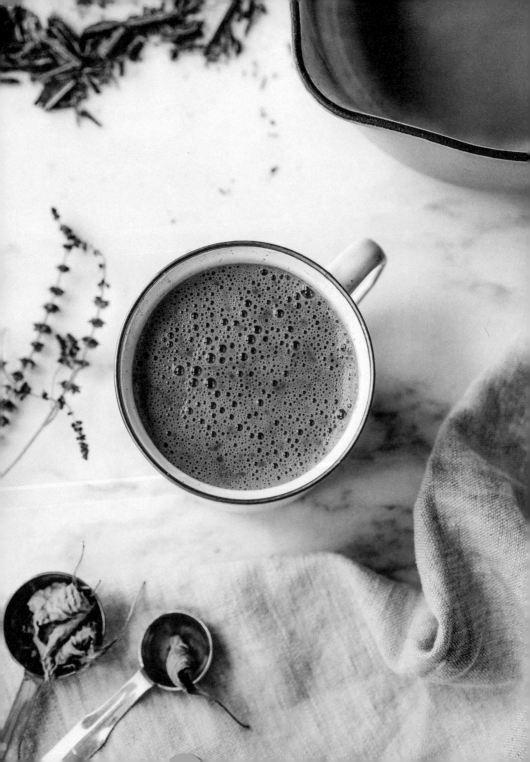

Mushroom Miso Broth

This warming and nourishing broth is one of my favorite ways to incorporate immune-supporting mushrooms into the kiddos' bellies. I serve this with soba noodles, topped with shaved carrots, toasted sesame seeds, and sliced scallions

Makes 4 servings

In a large pot or Dutch oven, heat the olive oil over medium heat. Add the garlic, ginger, and onion and sauté until the onion becomes translucent.

Add the stock, shiitakes, maitake, astragalus (if using), sea salt, and soy sauce. Stir and simmer for at least 45 minutes and up to 3 hours. The longer you simmer, the tastier the broth will become.

Add the miso paste and pinch of cayenne and stir. Serve the broth in a bowl and add noodles and toppings of your choice.

2 tablespoons olive oil

8 garlic cloves, minced

2 tablespoons minced fresh ginger

1 large onion, finely diced

8 cups vegetable stock or water

3 cups chopped shiitake mushrooms tops, fresh or dried

1 cup maitake, sliced

4 or 5 slices astragalus root (optional)

1 tablespoon sea salt, plus more to taste

2 tablespoons soy sauce

3 tablespoons white miso paste

Pinch of cayenne pepper

One package of buckwheat or soba noodles

Toasted sesame seeds, shaved carrots, sliced scallions for topping (optional)

Saved the Harvest for a Snowy Day

Why do we grow and prepare and harvest all year? Personal connection, cultivating plants to nurture the environment, and enduring the winter months. We squirrel away the energy of the sun in the form of dried herbs, canned produce, and food from our harvest. We store roots in the cellar and little chamomile blooms in jars to sustain our bodies, hearts, and minds through the winter.

Now is the time to pull out the elderberry jelly for a slice of sourdough bread and bring those summer moments to life on your winter table. Since living in the Midwest, as the sun wanes from the sky and the days grow darker, I lean heavily on those plants I harvest and store away. I get more creative to keep my spirit alive in the dark months as winter seems to drag on into January, February, and March. The holidays bring joy and light and energy and a spirit of celebration around the solstice, but what happens after that?

This is when I begin to incorporate warming herbal beverages and pull out lemon balm and tulsi tinctures from the shelves, St. John's wort oil rubbed on my skin after a shower, and flower essences to support my mood. I turn herbal oils into salves. It is when my connection to living plants is not as readily available that I yearn for it most. For you, it might be living in a city, where plants are harder to come by. We can turn to what we've preserved.

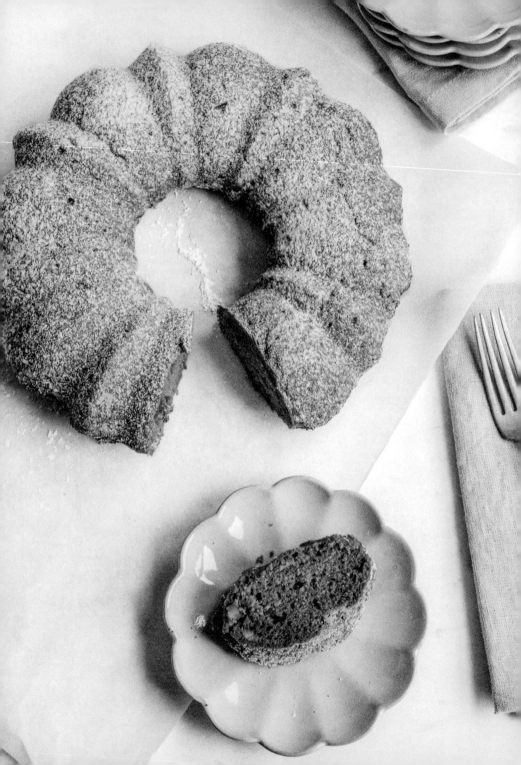

Persimmon, Walnut, and Chamomile Cake

In the winter months, I love infusing all our treats with herbal goodness, and cake is no exception. Chamomile infused into butter cuts its sometimes bitter flavor and adds a mellowness to this cake. Persimmons are a fruit I didn't grow up with, but I love to experiment with them when they arrive in the market come November.

Makes 1 (10-inch) Bundt cake

Preheat the oven to 325°F. Grease and flour a 9- to 10-inch Bundt pan.

In a large bowl, sift together the flour, cinnamon, baking soda, and salt. In a small saucepan, melt the butter and stir in the dried chamomile. Let sit for 5 minutes. Stir the butter, persimmon pulp, oil, honey or sugar, and eggs into the flour mixture just until incorporated. Fold in the chopped walnuts.

Pour the batter into the prepared pan, smoothing the top, and bake in the oven for 45 to 50 minutes, or until a toothpick comes out clean. Transfer to a wire rack and let cool. Dust with confectioners' sugar before serving, if desired.

3 cups all-purpose flour

1 teaspoon ground cinnamon

1 teaspoon baking soda

½ teaspoon kosher salt

½ cup (1 stick) salted butter

2 tablespoons dried chamomile

2 cups pureed persimmon pulp

½ cup olive oil

2 cups honey or sugar

3 large eggs

1 cup chopped walnuts, toasted

All-purpose flour, for dusting pan

Confectioners' sugar, for dusting (optional)

Après Dinner Tea

A digestif is an after-dinner drink that aids digestion, calms the stomach, and opens conversation and connection. This tea features carminative and nervines to help one digest both food and information and relax.

2 grams dried chamomile

0.5 grams dried orange peel

1 gram fennel seed

1 gram dried apple mint, spearmint, peppermint, or monarda

Cinnamon stick (optional)

4 cups boiling water

Honey

Makes 4 servings

Combine the herbs and cinnamon stick (if using) in a heatproof bowl. Cover with boiling water and steep for 10 minutes. Strain the tea, stir in a dollop of honey, and enjoy.

Elderberry Hot Toddy

A hot toddy is traditional when someone is feeling symptoms of a cold coming on, using hot water, sometimes tea, and a dash of whiskey. This recipe uses the immune-supporting elderberry syrup for more herbal support and a little sweetness.

1 tablespoon Elderberry Syrup (page 232)

1½ cups boiling water

Orange slice

1 ounce whiskey (optional)

Makes 1 serving

Pour the elderberry syrup into a mug, add the boiling water, and stir. Add a slice of orange and dash of whiskey (if using).

Calendula and Cardamom Granola

Granola is one of my favorite recipes for breakfast or a snack, or to eat on hikes. This simple recipe is made delicious with calendula petals dried from the summer harvest.

3 cups rolled oats

½ cup chopped pecans or walnuts

¼ cup sunflower seeds

½ teaspoon ground cinnamon

¼ teaspoon ground cardamom

½ teaspoon sea salt

¼ cup olive oil

½ cup honey or maple syrup

¼ cup dried calendula petals

Makes 6 to 8 servings

Preheat the oven to 325°F. Line a large baking sheet with parchment paper.

In a large bowl, mix together the rolled oats, pecans, sunflower seeds, cinnamon, cardamom, and salt.

In a small bowl, mix the olive oil and honey until blended well. Stir the wet ingredients into the dry ingredients and mix until well incorporated. Spread the granola mixture evenly in a single layer on the prepared baking sheet.

Bake for 20 minutes, or until golden brown, turning the baking sheet halfway through. Remove from the oven, sprinkle the calendula flowers on top, and let cool. Store in an airtight container or jar for up to one week. Serve over yogurt and top with elderberry jelly (page 231).

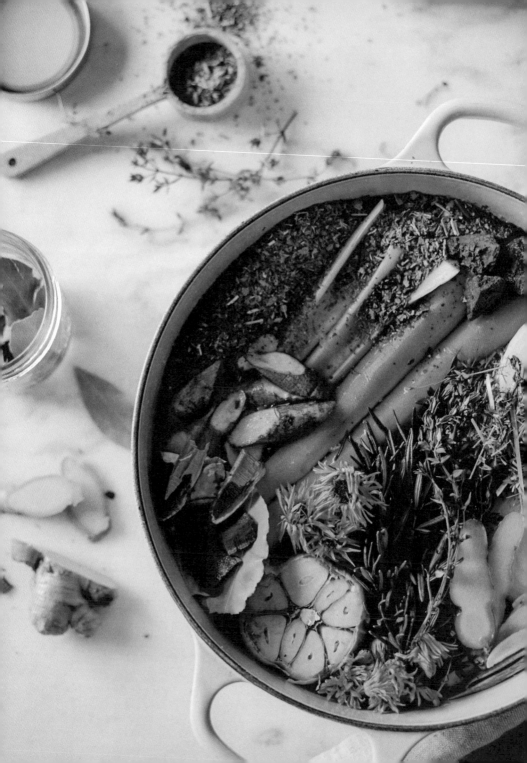

Herbal Bone Broth

Broth is a perfect way to make use of the odds and ends, to take the bones, the scraps, and turn them into nourishment and a potent medicine for winter. Broths are warming and nutritive. They can be used to cook rice, grains, soups, or enjoyed as a cupful on their own. This broth is full of herbal and immune supports as well. I save valuable cooking scraps and bones from roasted chicken in the freezer to make a batch. The scraps hold nutritious and flavorful parts; I include onion skins, leeks, celery, garlic skins, carrot peels and tops, mushroom stems, scallion tops, and herb stems.

4 carrots

1 whole shallot or leek

1 head of garlic

2-inch piece of ginger, sliced

¼ cup apple cider vinegar

2 fresh rosemary sprigs

5 fresh thyme sprigs

3 or 4 reishi mushroom slices

4 chaga mushroom chunks

2 to 3 tablespoons dried nettle

2 to 3 tablespoons dried oat straw

3 tablespoons chopped burdock root

2 tablespoons dried calendula flowers

4 or 5 dried astragalus slices

1 tablespoon dried sage

Kosher salt

3 celery stalks

1 whole onion

4 lbs of beef bones or a whole chicken carcass

Makes 12 servings

Combine all the ingredients in a large Dutch oven or stockpot. Add water to cover the ingredients, about 12 cups of water. Turn the heat to medium and bring to a boil, uncovered. Once it reaches a boil, turn down the heat to low and simmer, covered, for at least 4 hours and up to 8 hours, checking and replenishing the water as it evaporates. Once the broth is thick, remove from the heat. Let cool, then strain the mixture through a fine-mesh strainer, discarding the bones and composting the plant material. Pour into jars and refrigerate for up to four days.

Chamomile and Astragalus Moon Milk

Astragalus is an antiviral and adaptogenic herb that can be taken long-term as a tonic. I love to add it in soups and broths all winter long, as astragalus in the fall and early winter supports immunity. Astragalus also has an affinity with the respiratory system, fortifying the lungs. Note that astragalus should not be used in acute infections, as it can feed illness, according to traditional Chinese medicine, and is best used to support immune and respiratory function. Chamomile is an anti-inflammatory, nervine, and antimicrobial herb gentle enough for little ones. A cup of chamomile tea before bed can ease anyone into a space of calm and rest.

1 cup milk of your choice (I prefer oat milk)

2 teaspoons dried chamomile buds, or 1 chamomile tea bag

2 or 3 astragalus root slices

1 teaspoon honey, or more to taste

1 teaspoon ghee

Pinch of kosher salt

Makes 1 serving

Bring your milk almost to a boil in a saucepan set over medium heat. Add the chamomile and astragalus and turn down the heat to maintain a gentle simmer for 3 to 5 minutes. Remove from the heat, cover with a lid, and infuse for 5 to 10 minutes, leaving it longer for a stronger brew. Strain the milk through a mesh sieve into a blender and add the honey, ghee, and salt. Blend until frothy and well blended. Serve at once and snuggle in.

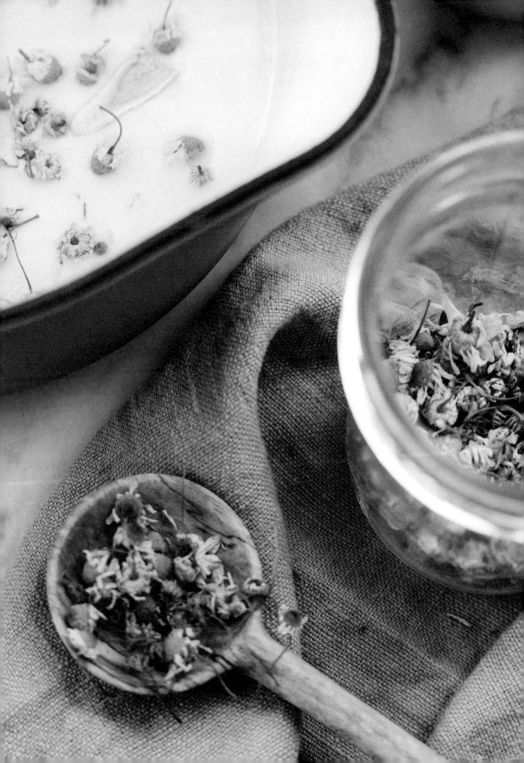

Calendula Whipped Body Butter

This simple three-ingredient body butter comes together from the calendula-infused oil made in the late summer. It is a perfect remedy while indoors during the winter months. With the dry heat of a wood stove and the cold winter air, my skin thirsts for moisture and hydration.

Body butters have a thicker consistency than lotion and go on the skin more smoothly than salves. Here I use a kitchen scale for measurements and make sure I have clean containers on hand. Repurposed jars and tins work well.

150 grams shea butter or mango butter

50 grams calendula-infused oil

5 grams jojoba oil

Optional: 5 drops essential oils

Makes 4 (2-ounce) jars or 8 ounces

Add the shea butter and calendula and jojoba oils to a double boiler, melt to combine into a liquid. Remove from heat and put in the refrigerator for an hour to cool. Add cooled mixture into a stand mixer or larger bowl with hand mixer or an immersion blender, whip the butter until it begins to form peaks, scraping down the sides of the bowl often. Add the essential oils if using and continue to mix until well blended and whitish, with a soft whipped consistency, about 10 minutes. Using a silicone spatula, spoon your butter into clean and dry containers to store. You don't want to introduce any water into this mixture as it can cause it to spoil. Use clean hands to apply the body butter to dry skin. It will keep for up to 6 months (less time in warm conditions). You can also store it in the refrigerator to extend its shelf life.

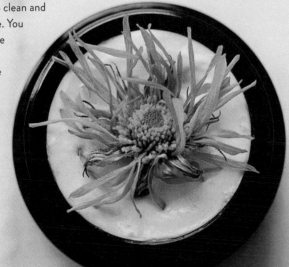

Lavender Linen Spray

In my mind, lavender is a perfect plant for the winter months. It stores well and brings deep peace; lavender is for dreaming a new world into being. In winter we hibernate, we slumber more, we dream. Lavender supports this. An herbal spray is a good alternative to herbal smoke to cleanse the energy of a space.

1½ ounces vodka

20 drops lavender essential oil

Makes 1 (8-ounce) spray bottle

Combine the vodka, essential oil, and 1½ ounces water in an amber spray bottle, shake to mix, and use to freshen sheets, pillows, clothes, and to cleanse the energy of your space.

Floor Cleansers

The floor is the root of our home. Like the ritual of foot baths to cleanse our personal energy, we can use herbs and plants to bless, clean, and utter spells of protection around our homes. Mint and yarrow are two herbs I enjoy using in this ritual.

Handful of dried herbs, such as mint and yarrow

1 quart boiling water

¼ cup herbal vinegar or distilled white vinegar

1 tablespoon borax powder

1-3 drops essential oil (optional)

Makes 1 quart (1 floor wash)

Steep a handful of dried herbs of your choice in the boiling water for 10 minutes, then strain and compost the herbs. Mix the "tea," vinegar, borax, and essential oil, if using, in a bucket, stir, and mop onto floors (be sure to sweep your floors first). Clean the surfaces, baseboards, thresholds, and sills of your home with a cloth imbued with the intention to clear your home of unwanted energy, washing away the residue of fights lingering in the halls and infusing your space with healing intention and protection. When you are done, toss the water out of your home, saying goodbye to the unwanted energy.

Nettle and Tulsi Chai

Makes 2 servings

Crush all the herbs and spices in a mortar and pestle. Pour them into a mason jar and cover with 8 to 12 ounces of boiling water. Steep between 1 and 4 four hours, then strain the mixture through a mesh sieve into a saucepan and heat over medium heat for five minutes or until warmed. Add honey or sugar to taste. Top with frothy steamed milk.

⅓ ounce dried nettle leaf

¼ ounce dried holy basil

1 cinnamon stick

1 inch piece ginger

6 cardamom pods

2 star anise pods

3 black peppercorns

3 cloves

1 bay leaf

½ teaspoon coriander seeds

Honey or sugar

Steamed milk (I like to use oat milk)

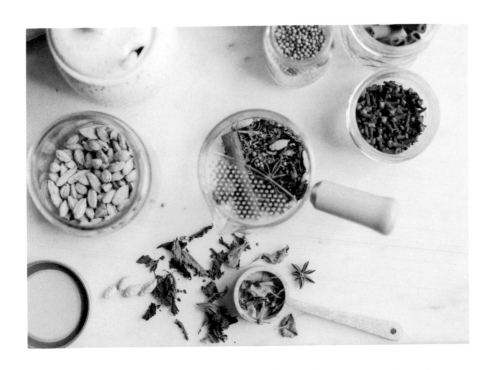

A Clean Slate

Around the turn of the calendar year, while we are still in winter hibernation, I like to make a ritual of cleaning our home. I'll freshen our space with herbal cleansing, sweeping out the corners of our home, my mind, and my heart. I'll open a window or two for cold, fresh air to blow through. I make the beds with fresh linens and prepare a linen spray with dried lavender or essential oils, wash the floor using herbs in the bucket, light an herbal bundle and carry it to every corner of our home while I recite a prayer as a way to cleanse the energy and bless each room with my intention. Herbs for protection at the front and back doors seal the energy and invite a sense of newness and calm, setting an intention for our home as we welcome the New Year.

Soup Joumou

Soup Joumou is more than a soup—it is food and ritual woven together in story keeping. A pot, a bowl, a vessel for remembrance and a helping of resistance. During colonial rule, this soup was made by the enslaved to be served only to enslavers. Today, it is made on January 1 throughout Haiti, served to Haitians in the street and made in diasporic homes worldwide to commemorate liberation. Soup Joumou or pumpkin soup is a reminder of strength, sovereignty, and independence over French colonialism, celebrated through food and sharing a meal. May Soup Joumou inspire us all to nourish ourselves and each other through our struggles, honor the ones who have come before us, and celebrate the strides and strength against oppression. This soup evokes the power of our food.

Makes 10 servings

Rinse the beef with water. Mix the épis, lime juice, and salt in a large bowl. Add the beef and coat it with the mixture. Let set for at least an hour or overnight in the refrigerator.

When the beef is ready, heat 6 cups of the broth in large stock pot over medium heat. Add the beef and beef bones, cover, and simmer until the meat has begun to cook. Add the squash, cover, and return to a simmer, cooking until the squash is softened, about 20 minutes. Using a slotted spoon, remove the squash and transfer it to a blender. Add 2 cups water and blend until smooth. Return the pureed squash to the pot and continue to cook. Add the potatoes, cabbage, carrots, onion, celery, leek, turnips, chile, cloves, minced garlic, onion powder, thyme, salt and pepper, olive oil, and the remaining 4 cups broth. Simmer until the vegetables are cooked, about 30 minutes. Stir in the noodles and cook, stirring occasionally, for another 10 minutes. If the soup is too thick, you can add extra broth or water. Remove thyme sprigs and serve.

1 beef shank

1 pound beef stew meat, cut into one-inch chunks

½ cup Épis (page 275)

Juice of 1 lime

2 teaspoons sea salt

10 cups beef broth

2 pounds kabocha or butternut squash, peeled, seeded, and cubed

2 large Yukon Gold potatoes, finely diced

½ head of cabbage

2 carrots, thinly sliced

1 medium yellow onion, diced

1 celery stalk, finely diced

1 leek, white part only, well washed and finely diced

2 small turnips, finely chopped

½ Scotch bonnet or habanero chile pepper

3 whole cloves

1 garlic clove, minced

1 teaspoon onion powder

1 fresh thyme sprig

Kosher salt and freshly ground black pepper

3 tablespoons olive oil

1 cup noodles, vermicelli, rigatoni, or elbow macaroni

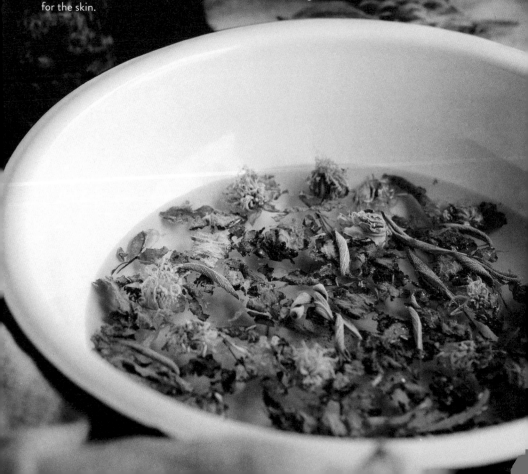

This is my go-to steam during the winter months to ease colds and issues in the respiratory system. Thyme is particularly helpful for drying, and sage is balancing.

2 tablespoons dried thyme

2 tablespoons dried monarda

2 tablespoons sage

2 or 3 drops of essential oil, such as eucalyptus, lavender, or sage (optional)

Makes 1 steam

Mix the dried herbs together in a heat-safe bowl. Pour boiling water over the herbs, add the essential oil, if using, and place the bowl at the edge of a table. Arrange a large towel over your head and the bowl and sit, inhaling the steam, for 5 to 15 minutes, allowing your nasal passages to drain. This is also nourishing for the skin.

Reseeding Our Future

"Another world is not only possible, she is on her way.
Maybe many of us won't be here to greet her, but on a quiet day,
if I listen very carefully, I can hear her breathing."

ARUNDHATI ROY

The new world will come from the ground up. The definition of the word *reparations* is to make amends for a wrong by helping those who have been harmed in some material and tangible way. The root of the word is "repair" or the Latin *reparae*, which translates to "make ready again." As my first and dear therapist, Hali, helped me learn, in relationships with other people, conflict can sting and it can hurt, but the most important aspect is the repair work put in. The communication, the care, and the tenderness given in its wake. The word *amend* means to make better by making minor changes, from the Latin *emendare*, "out of a fault." How can we use our hands and hearts to make whole our world that is damaged and injured? If the repair work is most important and most valuable, how do we begin?

What will we mend with the thread that binds us together, to our ancestors and our children? What future will we weave for tomorrow? It is my deepest hope that by encouraging intimate relationships with plants and the natural world, we will open portals to protect our kindred earth more fiercely.

Let's not allow the darkness of the past color the possibilities held within our present moment. Can we distill our pain down into a seed of wisdom to plant for future generations? Can we find the courage to meet ourselves in this moment? In our hearts and our collective action, we need to knit ourselves into reciprocity and accept interdependence as a vehicle for healing.

We need to nurture our soils, plant gardens to feed ourselves and each other, and tend to our local ecosystems. We need to heal ourselves and nurture our nervous systems so we can take clear, creative, and decisive action to heal the earth.

As I've begun to learn about cherishing bees as a part of my garden and my ecosystem, their organization provides inspiration for how we can look to work together as a whole. Bees work to serve the hive. An individual bee is an organism in and of itself, yet it works to support the superorganism that is the hive, the whole, the home. We can do the work in front of us, and that contributes to the wellness and harmony of the whole.

Healing doesn't need to happen in isolation, rather healing can be brought into the realm of the community. Let's gather around food, drink, and plants to nourish each other into wholeness. In the practice of building trust in one another, let us open our gardens, hearts, and homes in a spirit of shared humanity and kinship.

- Invite a neighbor into the garden to share a harvest of herbs, flowers, or just conversation.

- Lend a hand in a friend's garden.

- Make a cup of tea for an acquaintance from garden-grown herbs and lend an ear.

- Make a meal for a member of the community.

- Grow extra vegetables to donate to a local food pantry.

- Host a harvest meal or potluck.

- Start a local plant or seed swap.

- Plant trees and pollinator gardens.

- Host a circle to share climate griefs and anxiety around a heart-opening beverage.

- Invite friends into your kitchen to preserve the season's bounty and make herbal preparations.

- Host a land sit. Invite others to come and ground and root on your land and listen to the messages of the earth and the trees. Bring an offering and share what messages came through for the collective.

- Plan a dinner to gather community in a safe space for honest conversation, sharing food, grief, laughter, heartache, and joy.

As a society we should be thinking of doing the least amount of harm, asking questions: does this aid nature, is this extractive or reciprocal, and is it for the common good? These are the ways we open our hearts and homes to each other and the earth as kindred spirits.

What does a healed earth look like to you? What does a healed and whole version of yourself feel like if you were to experience it in your body? What steps can you take toward creative expressions of service to the earth and sovereignty? Nourish the vision your heart holds for your community and our earth.

Acknowledgments

I want to acknowledge this Earth we all call home, which shelters and feeds us, and brings us joy with its spring blossoms. To the water that we share and to the soil that feeds us and where we will all return to one day. Even when I have fear in my heart and words are caught in my throat, the way the sunlight hits my face and the ever-changing clouds float across the sky helps me remember why I'm grateful to be alive. Earth imbues me with the courage to live my most authentic self, in turn I have a fierce call to protect and fight for its survival.

To the plants who reached out to me—rosemary, lemon balm, elderflower—whose scents and smells and delights called me in to listen more deeply to the Earth and myself. On this plant path, my life diverged in ways I could have never imagined. I am indebted to you.

To my ancestors who have found homes in the stars. Your lives, journeys, and experiences have brought me to where I stand. Your exquisitely complicated stories, known and unknown, live on in my bones.

To my husband and partner on this cosmic journey, AJ Morgan, who with humor, love, and unwavering service has helped me create the space and time during a global pandemic to write my first book. He helps me make my dreams come true and loves me through my errors and in my humanity. Your love has given me courage and strength to love myself. He has stepped in, stepped up in ways, seen and unseen, so I could bring this book into being. I'm forever grateful to you.

To my parents, Geraldine and Anthony Cook, who have cared for me through my early arrival to this earth, through accidents, and on simple days, too. They encourage me and have loved me fiercely every day since my first breath and remind me what it means to come home. I am lucky to know them.

To my children: Magnolia, my moon, and Griffin, my sun. You are why I use my voice; their mere existence brings a smile to my face and tears to my eyes daily because I am grateful to have been given the gift of being their mother. I am grateful to them for their patience and unwavering love and for giving me the space to write and create.

To the herbal community that I've come to know and love and learn from. I humble myself at the wisdom, lessons, and experience that plant people so graciously share in pursuit of healing. To my various herbal teachers, friends, and mentors from conferences, workshops, courses, and conversations about plants and to those who open their gardens, hearts, and minds to me—our connections are rooted.

To the voices in written works who

have provided me with ways out of my own darkness and into my own light: bell hooks, Robin Wall Kimmerer, Rebecca Solnit, Joanna Macy, Mary Oliver.

To local friends and creatives Fran Knapp, Karlee Mikkelson and Kirsten Layer. To Fran, for being a dear and trusted friend for ten years, it is a dream to have your hard work and amazing skills showcased in my book. I hope you continue to create because the world needs it. Kirsten, for her testing, her stellar taste buds and food knowledge, her gentle but necessary critiques that helped me bring my recipes to this book. To Karlee for helping me capture parts of my visions for this book that I could not do on my own. It takes a village. To that end, I'm grateful for our little town and community that steps in to help and give support and encouragement all along the way, often times no questions asked. It is here I call home and laid down my roots.

To my editor, Michele Eniclerico, whose belief in this vision, sharp mind, and kind demeanor have guided me as I've brought these words from the depth of my being. Writing doesn't come easy and the support is immeasurable.

To my agent, Julia Eagleton, who has become a trusted friend and champion on this writing path.

To my therapist, Travis, I wouldn't and couldn't have written a book without years of sessions with you. Working with you helps me in ways I don't have words for, but maybe for my next book.

References

Abu-Reidah, Ibrahim M., Rana M. Jamous, and Mohammed Saleem Ali-Shtayeh. "Phytochemistry, Pharmacological Properties and Industrial Applications of Rhus coriaria L. (Sumac): A Review." *Jordan Journal of Biological Sciences* 7(4): 233–44.

Albrecht, Glenn, Gina-Maree Sartore, Linda Connor, Nick Higginbotham, Sonia Freeman, Brian Kelly, Helen Stain, Anne Tonna, and Georgia Pollard. "Solastalgia: The Distress Caused by Environmental Change." *Australasian Psychiatry* 15, Suppl. 1 (2007): S95–98. https://doi.org/10.1080/10398560701701288.

Andreae, Christine. "Slave Medicine." Monticello. Accessed April 20, 2022. https://www.monticello.org/sites/library/exhibits/lucymarks/medical/slavemedicine.html.

Atwood, Margaret. *Bluebeard's Egg*. Toronto: McClelland & Stewart, 1983.

Barnett, Jon, Petra Tschakert, Lesley Head, and W. Neil Adger. "A Science of Loss." *Nature Climate Change* 6, no. 11 (October 2016): 97678.

Brown, Brené. *The Gifts of Imperfection*. Minneapolis: Hazelden Publishing, 2010.

Brown, Brené. *I Thought It Was Just Me: Women Reclaiming Power and Courage in a Culture of Shame.* New York: Gotham Books, 2007.

Burke, Marshall, Felipe González, Patrick Baylis, Sam Heft-Neal, Ceyen Baysan, Sanjay Basu, and Solomon Hsiang. "Higher Temperatures Increase Suicide Rates in the United States and Mexico." *Nature Climate Change* 8 (2018): 723–29.

Cardwell, Glenn, Janet F. Bornman, Anthony P. James, and Lucinda J. Black. "A Review of Mushrooms as a Potential Source of Dietary Vitamin D." *Nutrients* 10, no. 10 (2018):1498. https://doi:10.3390/nu10101498.

Comtesse, Hannah, Verena Ertl, Sophie M. C. Hengst, Rita Rosner, and Geert E. Smid. "Ecological Grief as a Response to Environmental Change: A Mental Health Risk or Functional Response?" *International Journal of Environmental Research and Public Health* 18, no. 2 (2021): 734. https://doi.org/10.3390/ijerph18020734.

Cunsolo, Ashlee, and Ellis R. Neville. "Ecological Grief as a Mental Health Response to Climate Change-Related Loss." *Nature Climate Change* 8 (April 2018): 275–81.

Cunsolo, Ashlee, Sherilee L. Harper, Kelton Minor, Katie Hayes, Kimberly G. William, and Courtney Howards. "Ecological Grief and Anxiety: The Start of a Healthy Response to Climate Change?" *The Lancet* 4, no. 7 (July 2020): E261–63. https://doi.org/10.1016/S2542-5196(20)30144-3.

Davis, Donald R., Melvin D. Epp, and Hugh D. Riordan. "Changes in USDA Food Composition Data for 43 Garden Crops, 1950 to 1999." *Journal of the American College of Nutrition* 23, no. 6 (2004):669–82. https://doi:10.1080/07315724.2004.10719409.

Davis, Natalie. *Ho-Chunk Plants: Indigenous Plants of Winnebago Reservation, Nebraska.* Winnebago, NE: Little Priest Tribal College, 2010.

Desbordes, Gaëlle, Tim Gard, Elizabeth A. Hoge, Britta K. Hölzel, Catherine Kerr, Sara W. Lazar, Andrew Olendzki, and David R. Vago. "Moving Beyond Mindfulness: Defining Equanimity as an Outcome Measure in Meditation and Contemplative Research." *Mindfulness* 6 (January 2014): 356–72. https://doi.org/10.1007/s12671-013-0269-8.

Easley, Thomas, and Steven Horne. *The Modern Herbal Dispensatory: A Medicine-Making Guide.* Berkeley, CA: North Atlantic Books, 2016.

Eisler, Riane. *The Chalice and the Blade: Our History, Our Future.* New York: Harper Collins, 1987.

Eisler, Riane, and Douglas P. Fry. *Nuturing Our Humanity: How Domination and Partnership Shape Our Brains, Lives and Future.* New York: Oxford University Press, 2019.

Elpel, Thomas J. *Botany in a Day: The Patterns Method of Plant Identification: An Herbal Field Guide to Plant Families of North America,* 6th ed. Pony, MT: HOPS Press, 2013.

Estés, Clarissa Pinkola. "Do Not Lose Heart, We Were Made for These Times." MoonMagazine.org. March 13, 2020.

Federici, Silvia. *Caliban and the Witch: Women, the Body, and Primitive Accumulation.* Brooklyn, NY: Autonomedia, 2004.

Fornace, Kimberly M., et al. "Association between Landscape Factors and Spatial Patterns of Plasmodium knowlesi Infections in Sabah, Malaysia." *Emerging Infectious Diseases* 22, no. 2 (2016): 201–9.

Foxx, Christine L., et al. "Effects of Immunization with the Soil-Derived Bacterium *Mycobacterium vaccae* on Stress Coping Behaviors and Cognitive Performance in a 'Two Hit' Stressor Model." *Front Physiology* 11 (January 2021). https://doi .org/10.3389/fphys.2020.524833.

Gardner, Zöe, and Michael McGuffin, eds. *American Herbal Products Association's Botanical Safety Handbook*. 2nd ed. Boca Raton, FL: CRC Press, 2013.

Grad, Frank P. "The Preamble of the Constitution of the World Health Organization." *Bulletin of the World Health Organization* 80, no. 12 (2002): 981–84.

Griffiths, Jay. "Daily Grace." Aeon. January 31, 2019. Accessed April 23, 2022. https://aeon.co/ essays/how-rituals-can-protect-life-with-a-petal-and-a-prayer.

Hall, Joan Wylie, ed. *Conversations with Audre Lorde*. Jackson: University Press of Mississippi, 2004.

Hamby, Erin Brooke. "The Roots of Healing: Archaeological and Historical Investigations of African-American Herbal Medicine." PhD diss., University of Tennessee, Knoxville, 2004. https://trace.tennessee.edu/utk_graddiss/4543.

Herb Society of America. *Calendula: An Herb Society of America Guide*. Kirkland, OH: Herb Society of America, 2007.

Herbal Academy. *Herbal First Aid: The Herbal Academy's Handbook of Herbal First Aid Recipes*. Bedford, MA: Herbal Academy, n.d.

Herbal Academy. *Herbal Skin Care*. Bedford, MA: Herbal Academy, n.d.

hooks, bell. *All About Love: New Visions*. New York, NY: Harper Collins, 2001.

hooks, bell. "Love as the Practice of Freedom." Chap. 20 in *Outlaw Culture: Resisting Representations*. New York: Routledge, 1994.

Hurston, Zora Neale. *Their Eyes Were Watching God*. London: Virago Press, 2018.

Judith, Anodea. *Eastern Body, Western Mind: Psychology and the Chakra System as a Path to the Self*. Berkeley, CA: Celestial Arts, 1996.

Kimmerer, Robin Wall. *Braiding Sweetgrass: Indigenous Wisdom, Scientific Knowledge, and the Teaching of Plants*. Minneapolis, MN: Milkweed Editions, 2013.

Kolk, Bessel Van Der. *The Body Keeps Score: Brain, Mind and Body in the Healing of Trauma*. New York, NY: Penguin Random House, 2014.

Korkmaz, Hasan. "Could Sumac Be Effective on COVID-19 Treatment?" *Journal of Medicinal Food* 24, no. 6 (June 2021):563–68. https://doi. org/10.1089/jmf.2020.0104.

Lee, Michele E. *Working the Roots: Over 400 Years of Traditional African-American Healing*. Oakland, CA: Wadastick Publishers, 2014.

Lon, Jonathan, and David Harmon. *Biocultural Diversity: Threatened Species, Endangered Languages*. Zeist, the Netherlands: WWF Netherlands, 2014.

Lorde, Audre. *Sister Outsider: Essays and Speeches*. Trumansburg, NY: Crossing Press, 1984.

Macy, Joanna. *World as Lover, World as Self: Courage for Global Justice and Ecological Renewal*. Berkeley, CA: Parallax Press, 2007.

Menakem, Resmaa. *My Grandmother's Hands: Racialized Trauma and the Pathways to Mending Our Hearts and Bodies*. Las Vegas: Central Recovery Press, 2017.

Penniman, Leah. *Farming While Black: Soul Fire Farm's Practical Guide to Liberation on the Land*. White River Junction, VT: Chelsea Green, 2018.

Phillips, Michael. *Mycorrhizal Planet: How Symbiotic Fungi Work with Roots to Support Plant Health and Build Soil Fertility*. White River Junction, VT: Chelsea Green, 2017.

Ray, Amit. *The Science of 114 Chakras in Human Body: A Guidebook*. Rishikesh, India: Inner Light, 2015.

Rilke, Rainer Maria. *Letters to a Young Poet*. New York: Penguin Classics, 2016.

Romm, Aviva. *Botanical Medicine for Women's Health.* 2nd ed. St. Louis, MO: Elsevier Health Sciences, 2017.

Roy, Arundhati. *The God of Small Things.* London: Fourth Estate, 1997.

Schafer, Patricia D. "A Manual of Cherokee Herbal Remedies: History, Information, Identification, Medicinal Healing." Master's thesis, Indiana State University, March 1993. Accessed April 23, 2022. https://files.eric.ed.gov/fulltext/ED396878.pdf.

Scheffer, Mechthild. *The Encyclopedia of Bach Flower Therapy,* trans. Walter C. Schell. Rochester, VT: Healing Arts Press, 1996.

Seca, Anna M. L., Alice Grigore, Diana C. G. A. Pinto, and Artur M. S. Silva. "The Genus *Inula* and Their Metabolites: From Ethnopharmacological to Medicinal Uses." *Journal of Ethnopharmacology* 154, no. 2 (June 2014): 286–310. https://doi.org/10.1016/j.jep.2014.04.010.

Singh, Ompal, Zakia Khanam, Neelam Misra, and Manoj K. Srivastava. "Chamomile (*Matricaria chamomilla* L.): An Overview." *Pharmacognosy Review* 5, no. 9 (January–June 2011): 82–95.

Smith, David G., et al. "Identification and Characterization of a Novel Anti-inflammatory Lipid Isolated from *Mycobacterium vaccae*, a Soil-Derived Bacterium with Immunoregulatory and Stress Resilience Properties." *Psychopharmacology (Berl)* 236, no. 5 (May 2019): 1653–70. https://doi.org/10.1007/s00213-019-05253-9.

Solnit, Rebecca. *Hope in the Dark: Untold Histories, Wild Possibilities.* New York: Nation Books, 2004.

Stansbury, Dr. Jill. *Neurology, Psychiatry, and Pain Management including Cognitive and Neurologic Conditions and Emotional Conditions.* Vol. 4 of *Herbal Formularies for Health Professionals.* White River Junction, VT: Chelsea Green, 2020.

Teplicki, Eric, Qianli Ma, David E. Castillo, Mina Zarei, Adam P. Hustad, Juan Chen, and Jei Li. "The Effects of *Aloe vera* on Wound Healing in Cell Proliferation, Migration, and Viability." *Wounds* 30, no. 9 (September 2018): 263–68.

Thomas-Stevenson, Bonnie. "Ozarkian and Haitian Folk Medicine." Webster University, 1991. Accessed April 23, 2022. http://faculty.webster.edu/corbetre/haiti-archive/msg03384.html.

Volpato, Gabriele, Daimy Godínez, Angela Beyra, and Adelaida Barreto. "Uses of Medicinal Plants by Haitian Immigrants and Their Descendants in the Province of Camagüey, Cuba." *Journal of Ethnobiology and Ethnomedicine* 5 (May 2009): 16. https://doi.org/10.1186/1746-4269-5-16.

Walker, Alice. *Living by the Word: Selected Writings, 1973–1987.* New York: Harcourt Brace, 1988.

Wisneski, Leonard A. *The Scientific Basis of Integrative Medicine.* 3rd ed. Boca Raton, FL: CRC Press, 2009.

Yang, Sarah. "Human Security at Risk as Depletion of Soil Accelerates, Scientists Warn." Berkeley News. May 7, 2015. Accessed April 23, 2022. https://news.berkeley.edu/2015/05/07/soil-depletion-human-security/.

Index

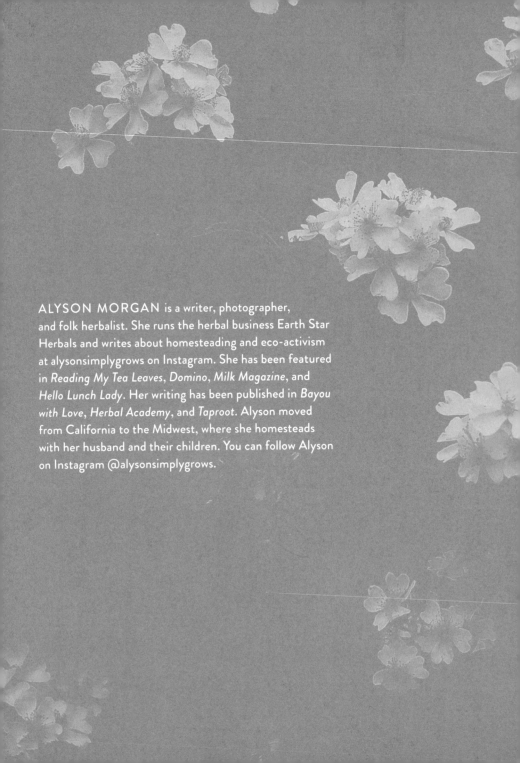

ALYSON MORGAN is a writer, photographer, and folk herbalist. She runs the herbal business Earth Star Herbals and writes about homesteading and eco-activism at alysonsimplygrows on Instagram. She has been featured in *Reading My Tea Leaves*, *Domino*, *Milk Magazine*, and *Hello Lunch Lady*. Her writing has been published in *Bayou with Love*, *Herbal Academy*, and *Taproot*. Alyson moved from California to the Midwest, where she homesteads with her husband and their children. You can follow Alyson on Instagram @alysonsimplygrows.